ENDO UNFILTERED

ENDO UNFILTERED

How to take charge of your endometriosis and PCOS

ERIN BARNETT

murdoch books
Sydney | London

Published in 2022 by Murdoch Books, an imprint of Allen & Unwin

Murdoch Books Australia
83 Alexander Street, Crows Nest NSW 2065
Phone: +61 (0)2 8425 0100
murdochbooks.com.au
info@murdochbooks.com.au

Murdoch Books UK
Ormond House, 26–27 Boswell Street, London WC1N 3JZ
Phone: +44 (0) 20 8785 5995
murdochbooks.co.uk
info@murdochbooks.co.uk

 A catalogue record for this book is available from the National Library of Australia

A catalogue record for this book is available from the British Library

ISBN 9 781 92261 609 8

Cover design by Alissa Dinallo
Text design by Susanne Geppert
Illustrations by Sarah McCoy
Cover photography © iStock

Typeset by Midland Typesetters, Australia
Printed and bound in Australia by Griffin Press

We acknowledge that we meet and work on the traditional lands of the Cammeraygal people of the Eora Nation and pay our respects to their elders past, present and future.

10 9 8 7 6 5 4 3 2 1

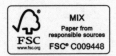 The paper in this book is FSC® certified. FSC® promotes environmentally responsible, socially beneficial and economically viable management of the world's forests.

To Nanna, my role model and best friend from the beginning. You're the OG endo sufferer in my life (it's kind of your fault that I have it!) and I love you so much.

Contents

Oh, damn

You've opened this book.

I'm sorry.

Don't get me wrong, this is a bloody great book and there's so much in here that you're going to laugh at or find interesting and helpful. But the fact you went looking for a book like this in the first place means one of three things:

1. You follow me on social media or know me from TV and wanted to check this out (thanks, babe!).

2. Someone you care about is suffering from endometriosis (aka, endo) and/or PCOS and you want to help them. If that's the case, good on you!

3. Or, the most likely option . . .
You've got one (or maybe both) of the disorders I just mentioned, and you're here for help, advice and/or comfort. I'm so glad we found each other.

If you know me from a TV show or two, you might be thinking, *Does Erin really know enough about endo and PCOS to write a whole book?* The answer to that question is a hard YES! In fact, I've been preparing for this book ever since my reproductive organs first twitched into action. Because I like to overdeliver, I've got endo *and* PCOS. They don't often go together, but when they do, let me tell you, they're best freakin' buddies.

To date, I've had 16 surgeries to treat my PCOS and endo. From the age of 14, various parts of my insides have been sliced, stitched, burned, removed and unstuck, again and again. Cysts have burst inside me like New Year's fireworks. I've had an ovary removed. I've experienced the intensity of medically induced menopause. And, through it all, I've bled. A lot. From my local supermarket to the South African jungle; if I've been there, I've probably bled there (fellow endo warriors know).

Physically, mentally and emotionally, the past six years have been especially relentless, but that was just my life. Sitting down to type out a timeline of all the procedures and treatments I've had for this book was the first time I was able to really reflect on it all. In some ways, looking at it listed in black and white has helped me see things from an outside perspective. Now that I have, it's wild to see that the cycle of surgery, pain, pills, bleeding and more surgery hasn't stopped. When I look at that timeline on pages 88–90, I think, *Oh, wow! No wonder I feel like an old nanna even though I'm only 26. Look at everything my body has been through.* All while trying to juggle work, romantic relationships and a social life (and, more recently, a public one).

The truth is, a lot of what I've been through has really sucked. Some of my experiences were so upsetting they inspired me to study nursing so I could make sure other people don't have to go through the things I did. If you're a fellow sufferer, the reality is that things are probably going to suck for you too, sometimes. In fact, let's hit pause to look at this extremely scientific diagram, which accurately illustrates how life with endo has been for me.

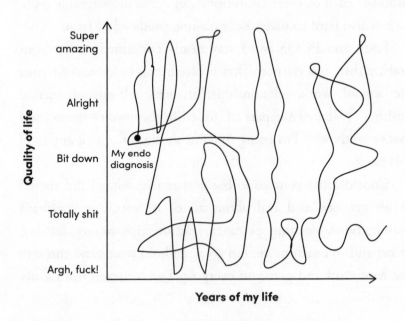

As you can see, calling life with endo a roller coaster is a massive understatement. It's more like a runaway train with a rocket strapped to it. But writing this book is a way for me to turn my negative experiences into stories that can empower sufferers and empathisers, and put them on a better path to dealing with the challenges they're facing. Being able to do this makes me grateful for the ride I've been on.

It's not always possible to see endo on a scan, but the pain is beyond real and it is definitely not 'normal'.[1] If you've got endo or PCOS, then – through no fault of your own – you've got a condition with no known cause and no known cure. Most doctors don't know enough to treat either effectively, so you're bound to hit roadblocks and be frustrated. You're also likely to feel dismissed and misunderstood a lot of the time because although each of these conditions can cause unbelievable pain, each is also hard to diagnose, measure, predict and treat.

Endo and PCOS won't stay neatly contained within your body, either. No chance. They'll bleed into every area of your life: school, work, relationships, finances, self-esteem, mental health . . . There's no part of your life they won't touch, and that's exactly why I'm going to come at them from all angles in this book.

Consider me your endo big cyst-er (see what I did there!) as we get raw and real about all of it: surgeries, awkward examinations, bleeding, pain, sex, relationships, money, fertility, career and so much more. I'm going to hold your hand through the hard stuff and give you every tip I've collected during my

---

1 When I use the word 'normal' in this book, I don't want you to think you're not normal (what is normal anyway?). I mean it in the context of the average person not experiencing the effects of endometriosis or PCOS.

journey to make your road less bumpy. If there's a young person in your life who is living with endo or PCOS, hand them this book and I'll talk them through it. Fair warning: there's the odd swear word here and there, as well as some real talk about sex, but I guarantee young people hear worse at school. And trust me, if they have endo or PCOS, it's nothing they can't handle.

I want to be clear about one thing up front: I didn't write this book to promise you that you'll be fine, or to say, 'I'm going to get you through this.' I do believe you'll be alright, but I'm not a magician. I can't make things okay for you, take away your pain or cure you. Endo and PCOS are not the easiest conditions to control. What I *can* do is give you a raw and real account of how things have been for me so you get a heads-up about what you may encounter. I can also introduce you to some new ways of thinking, as well as a friendly nudge of encouragement to take charge of the things that ARE in your control.

I'll be talking about a few not-so-great experiences I've had – most of which I really hope you *don't* have. A lot of it isn't pretty, but here's how I see it: when you go into situations with your eyes wide open, you're better prepared to deal with them. There's power in that.

That's why I've been so excited to write this book; I want more of us to hold the power when it comes to our health and our lives. I want you to read this book and think, *Now that I know it can be different, I'm going to ask these questions next time I see the doctor.* Or, *I'm going to insist we investigate until we find out what's really going on with me.* I'm going to help you get your way with your GP – I want you to feel more confident going into your appointments and surgeries, and when approaching any medical professional for that matter.

Every morning, when I pick up my phone, there are tonnes of messages on my social media from endo sufferers looking for reassurance, support or advice. I get DMs from women in pain who are unsure of what to do next, frustrated because some surgery or treatment hasn't worked, at the end of their rope with pain, or delighted because – finally – something HAS worked! These messages come from all over the world – the Netherlands, India, the UK, Australia, America . . .

No matter where we live, we're bound together by our shared experiences of not being taken seriously and having our pain dismissed by people who don't know or want to know. Although I talk about 'women' being endo and PCOS sufferers throughout this book because women are the people largely affected by these diseases, it's important to also remember that there are plenty of people in the LGBTQ+ community – transgender men or individuals who are non-binary – who may not identify as women, but who still have to live with endo or PCOS. It makes these diseases even harder for them to live through, and can add layers of psychological trauma to an already shit situation.

Too many of the people I hear from are stumbling along this journey blindfolded. Some want to know whether they should have the surgery their doctor is recommending. They are scared to undergo the procedure but they are scared not to because they can't face another decade of pain. I tell them surgery is nothing compared to suffering for so long because that's what I believe.

The pain and frustration in these messages is so familiar to me – I know it and I *feel* it. I screenshot the messages I need to reply to so I can respond that evening, and then I get up, get ready and go about my day. But, during the day, those messages swim around in my brain. I'll be at work or doing a food shop thinking, *How can I help that person?* Now, I can tell them to read this book because I'm about to answer the questions I get asked again and again, and so much more.

Whenever I mention a certain drug or treatment I've tried and talk about my experience with it, my comments blow up with people accusing me of promoting that thing and being paid to push it out to my followers. So, let me also be clear about this: the point of this book is NOT to advocate for any surgeries or treatments. Obviously, I have opinions about things that have been done to or put inside my body, and it's my absolute right to share those. But doing that doesn't mean I'm promoting a certain pill, pain treatment or product. I'm simply telling you everything I've tried – not so you go out and do the same, just so you have more information.

If you want to take my experiences and give certain things a try for yourself, go for it. I encourage you to make choices that feel right for your body and your life when you have all the relevant information. I'm giving you my story in full with the hope it leaves you better informed, and with a fire in your belly to stand up for yourself.

I'm so glad you're coming on this ride with me. Buckle up, and be prepared to laugh, cry and feel 1000 emotions over the next few hundred pages. If I've done my job well, by the end of this book, you'll be standing up for yourself like a champ and reeling off medical terminology like an expert – minus the medical degree.

Speaking of medical degrees, you'll be hearing from Dr Tom Manley in on page 63. He's one of Australia's leading obstetricians and surgical gynaecologists. He also happens to be my favourite doctor, and the surgeon who has been treating me for the past few years. He's a legend when it comes to laparoscopic surgery, endometriosis, PCOS, pelvic pain, cysts, fibroids . . . but the thing I love most about Dr Manley is that he's on a hunt for real solutions. I'm excited for him to be a part of this book and give us his medical perspective. He's smart as anything, knows his shit and talks the way I talk – like a real person, just way more professional.

I know that it's easy to say, 'We're all in this together', but day-to-day, a lot of what we face, we go through on our own – hunched over at work, cramping in the shower, crying on the couch. Just promise me that you'll remember one thing: as alone as you might feel in those moments, there are SO many people experiencing the same thing in that moment, too. I'm going to help you connect with them, if you haven't already, because that community really is with you, and so am I.

As each of us finds our own way through this, it's up to us to turn on a light for those coming behind us. This book is my way of doing that. My hope is that there will be a lot in here that stops you and makes you think, *Thank God she's talking about this*, because often when we go into a doctor's office and have a procedure explained or a diagram shown to us, that language and those images don't help us to understand how these things are going to *feel* in our bodies. They don't paint an accurate picture of the *experience* of living with these conditions. Let's fix that now.

BONUS!!
Your endo and PCOS cheatsheet

I gotta be honest, when it comes to reading books about health or real-life stuff, I'm definitely that person skipping through the pages to find the one thing I'm looking for. You're probably here because you need an answer or advice about a particular issue, and if you're anything like me, you need it NOW. That's exactly why I've created this handy li'l cheatsheet for you.

I've included things I think you'll be looking for and where to find them. But here's the deal: after you've found the answer and you've dealt with whatever it is you're facing right now, go back and read more. There's a tonne of other info in this book you'll probably find useful. You don't have to read it front to back. There won't be a test after. I don't care how you read it as long as it helps you. Stash the book next to the toilet or by your bed, and it will be waiting for you the next time you need an answer, an idea of what to ask at your next appointment, or a reminder that you're not alone in this.

Help, Erin! I need to know . . .

How to deal with endo pain
69

How to stop endo from ruining my relationship
147

What to do about painful sex
155

What to expect at my internal ultrasound
40

What to expect at my surgery
111

What to pack for my hospital stay
114

How to find out if I have PCOS
25

Where to find more helpful information
210

I also get asked about my current relationship,
so if you want that info, see page **141**.

And for the latest in my surgery saga, see page **201**.

1

xxx

Meet endometriosis and PCOS

Being blindsided sucks, especially when that thing you didn't see coming is something big. Without a doubt, the most traumatic experiences I've had throughout this whole endo/PCOS journey have happened because I didn't know enough about a situation going into it – be it a procedure, a surgery or my rights as a patient. So many things were a surprise to me, and not the good kind. That's why, in this chapter, I'm going to lay a rock-solid foundation for you by sharing some facts about endometriosis and PCOS. I'll also give you an idea of how their effects can play out in real life.

The thing is, when doctors need to tell a patient they have a disease that has no cure – like endo – it's tempting for them to either 'dumb down' the full explanation of the condition or downplay the long-term challenges. That way, they won't over-whelm the patient. In a way, I understand this. Hearing that you have a condition that may require many medical interventions throughout your life is a heavy thing. A doctor might sugar-coat some of the details if they aren't sure you can handle it – especially if you are young. And you know what? Maybe you *will* have a hard time hearing the news. Maybe you will be sad or angry, or both. But that's okay. It doesn't mean you don't deserve the full picture, and it doesn't mean you aren't strong enough to deal with the things that are going to come your way. You are.

Trust me, having a good understanding of what *can* happen will make your life easier in the long run. That way, anything that *doesn't* happen is a bonus. On the flip side, thinking something isn't such a big deal and then finding out it's so much worse than you could have imagined is not fun. So, let's be real about the fact that endo and PCOS are conditions that have the *potential* to impact your happiness, health, quality of life, relationships and fertility, not to mention your finances, since you can rack up tens of thousands of dollars in healthcare costs paying for treatments. I'm not saying they definitely will; I'm just saying they can.

On a more positive note, the spectrum of endo experiences is vast, and where you fall on it is anyone's guess. Some women can have what's known as 'silent endo' where they never suffer symptoms (though I've never met someone who falls into this category),[2,3] some will have mild symptoms while some will suffer a lot. Research even tells us that there are people who have

---

2 Endometriosis New Zealand.
3 *Journal of Assisted Reproduction and Genetics.*

had their endo go away without treatment.[4] To be honest, this type of person sounds like an endo unicorn to me – a myth that exists to give the rest of us hope, but if they're out there, I'm honestly so happy for them!

All I know for sure is that you deserve to have all the information laid out in front of you. These days, when I'm with a doctor or surgeon, I say, 'Tell me everything. I want to know every last detail of what is going to happen during the procedure and what might happen after it.' I prefer to go into every situation with my eyes wide open – fully prepared for what *could* be. If I don't experience some of the negative things they warned me about, that's a huge win. If I do, well, at least I saw them coming.

Endometriosis

Let's start with a deep dive on this bad boy. It's pronounced *end-oh-mee-tree-oh-sis* – endo for short – just in case you aren't sure. My nanna was diagnosed back in the sixties and still struggles to say it, and I definitely tripped over it for a while myself. As far as diseases go, endo is even more mysterious than its pronunciation. There's no known cause, though there seems to be a link between a family history of endo (true in my case) and also between how young you are when you start your period; endo sufferers often start their periods earlier – often around 11 or 12. Short menstrual cycles and heavy or long periods that last for more than seven days also seem

---

4 The Women's (The Royal Women's Hospital, Victoria, Australia).

to be a factor, but again there are no clear answers.[5] If you're wondering what you did to cause your endo, the answer is nothing! None of this is your fault.

Endometriosis is divided into four stages. When you get an official diagnosis, your doctor should tell you which stage you have. If they don't, well, now you know to ask!

Stage 1 endometriosis (minimal):[6] Typically small patches of endo, surface lesions or inflammation on or around organs in the pelvic cavity.

Stage 2 endometriosis (mild): Endo is more extensive than in stage 1; it might have infiltrated the organs in the pelvis in a limited way. However, there isn't much scarring or many adhesions (we'll talk about adhesions in a minute).

Stage 3 endometriosis (moderate): Endo might be more widespread and starting to infiltrate pelvic organs, peritoneum (pelvic side walls) or other structures more. There is also scarring and adhesions.

Stage 4 endometriosis (severe): This is where endo is referred to as 'infiltrative' – when it affects many pelvic organs and the ovaries. Severe endo can distort your internal anatomy because parts of you can get stuck together by adhesions (the 'frozen pelvis' we talk about on the next page). This is my one, baby!

---

5 Australian Institute of Health and Welfare.
6 Endometriosis New Zealand.

Bizarrely, these stages don't necessarily correlate to how much pain someone has. You could have stage 1 endo yet be in total agony, while another woman has stage 3 but is out there living life relatively pain free. Remember, endo follows no rules!

In addition to those four stages there are also three different *types* of endo.

1. **Superficial peritoneal endometriosis:** This is the least severe form of endometriosis. The endo lesions grow on the surface of the peritoneum, the thin membrane that lines the pelvis and abdomen. Eighty per cent of sufferers have this type of endometriosis.

2. **Cystic ovarian endometriosis (or endometrioma):** The endo can implant on one or both ovaries, and also deep inside the ovaries, creating dark fluid-filled cavities inside them known as endometriomas or 'chocolate cysts' (ewww! Don't love that name).

3. **Deep infiltrative endometriosis (DIE):** This type of endo doesn't just grow on the surface of the organs in the pelvic area, it infiltrates more than 5 millimetres into the membrane and grows *inside* organs. Because DIE can create so much inflammation and scarring, it can cause something called 'frozen pelvis', which is when organs get stuck together, often in the wrong positions.

Researchers have known about these different types of endo for a decade, but it's only in the last five years that they've become more widely acknowledged and researched.[7] I'm pretty sure I have all three, but I've never been told this. It would be worth knowing though, because researchers believe different types of endo respond to different treatments. We'll explore this more in Chapter 3.

If you've been diagnosed with endo, or you think you might have it and you live in Australia, Endometriosis Australia's website is a great one to look at because they've got all sorts of Australia-specific info that will be useful. If you live in another country, I definitely recommend checking out the official endometriosis sites where you are – I've collected a few links at the back of this book to get you started.

One of the things I love on Endometriosis Australia's site is their 10 key facts about endo.[8] These facts do double duty because they also bust the most common myths about endo.

10 Key Facts

1. There is no cure for endometriosis.
2. Teenagers are NOT too young to have endometriosis.
3. Hysterectomy is NOT a cure for endometriosis.
4. Endometriosis can NOT be prevented.
5. Endometriosis does NOT always cause infertility.
6. Period pain is NOT normal.
7. Getting pregnant will NOT cure endometriosis.

---

7   *The Guardian.*
8   Endometriosis Australia.

8. Endometriosis can only be correctly diagnosed through surgical intervention.
9. Pain levels are NOT related to the extent of the disease.
10. Endometriosis is NOT an STI. You can NOT catch it.

What the hell is it?

I wish I knew how to fully answer this question; I wish someone – anyone – did! In a nutshell, endometriosis is a disease where tissue that is very similar to endometrial tissue, the membrane lining the uterus, implants itself *outside* of the uterus on other parts of your body and grows there. Notice how I said it's 'VERY SIMILAR' to endometrial tissue? That's because endometriosis is NOT the same as this lining, it's just very similar. Be warned, people online will have an absolute hissy fit if you say it's the same. (That's a little tip I've learned the hard way.)

Let's run through how periods work real quick because, trust me, it's helpful. In a 'normal' menstrual cycle, when estrogen and progesterone levels increase, they trigger the endometrial tissue that lines the uterus (aka womb) to thicken up so it's nice and cushy if and when an egg arrives.

High estrogen levels tell the pituitary gland in your brain to release a luteinising hormone, which makes one of your ovaries release an egg (they take turns and alternate egg delivery every month). That egg then travels down the fallopian tube, drops into the womb and implants into that cushy lining. If that egg wasn't fertilised when it was going down the fallopian tube, the body kicks into action to clear the decks.

The levels of progesterone in the bloodstream drop way off, and this leads to the shedding of that thick endometrial lining. The lining, along with the unused egg, will then fall away from the walls of the uterus and start flowing out of your body and into your pad, tampon, menstrual cup or period undies. The period cramps you feel are your body's way of shaking that lining free. Light cramping and aching during your cycle is part of your body's process. But, as we covered in the 10 facts about endo, pain – actual pain that doubles you over and takes away from the quality of your life – is not normal.

With endometriosis, unlike the healthy endometrial tissue that grows where it's supposed to and follows orders each cycle, the tissue does whatever the hell it wants and grows wherever it damn well pleases – lungs, abdomen, brain, spine . . . it follows zero rules. In my body, endo has grown on my bowel, bladder, uterus, ovaries and on my fallopian tubes (yay, me!). Why does it spread around the body, you ask? Again, nobody knows! See, I told you I'd give it to you straight. I'm not even pretending I can answer that one.

I often refer to endo as 'leeches' because I've seen images taken inside me during surgery, and that's what it looks like: those blood-sucking leeches you get from wading in a creek.

The crazy thing about endometriosis is that because it's SIMILAR to (remember, NOT the same as) the lining of your uterus, it reacts to hormones in the same way as that cushy lining does. So, when those hormone levels drop off and your womb starts aching and cramping in preparation to shed, so will your endo. When the lining of your uterus falls away and starts bleeding, so will your endo. But unlike the blood and tissue in the uterus, which has a clear exit route out of your body thanks to the vagina, the blood from your endo doesn't have anywhere to go, so it stays inside you. And if you happen to have endometriosis growing inside an ovary, which is pretty common, that ovary will fill with blood when the endo bleeds, resulting in a type of ovarian cyst called an endometrioma. That's a fancy name for what is basically a sac of old blood. Nice, right?

This powerful hormonal response is the reason periods can be extra painful for endo sufferers – they aren't just experiencing period cramps and bleeding in their uterus and vagina, they're experiencing it EVERYWHERE their endo is growing.

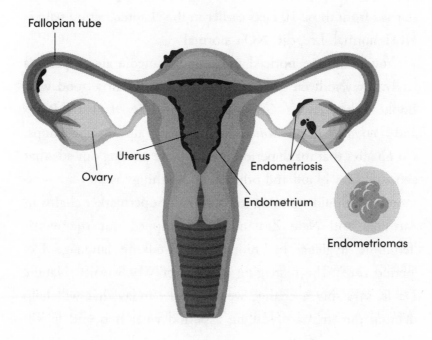

Fallopian tube

Uterus

Ovary

Endometriosis

Endometrium

Endometriomas

How do you know if you have endo?

Great question! Let's look at the most common symptoms:

- Pain (super-vague, right?)
- Heavy menstrual bleeding (also pretty vague)
- Bleeding between periods (okay, we can work with this one, it's a little more specific)
- Lethargy (*annnd* we're back to vague. Who isn't tired these days?)
- Reduced fertility (*sigh* vague *and* also something you're probably not going to even realise for years).

Looking at this list, it's easy to see why a lot of endo symptoms get thrown in the same bucket as regular period pain. But, as we learned from those 10 facts earlier in the chapter, period pain is NOT normal. I repeat, NOT normal.

You may have noticed more in the media about periods lately. They've been getting some attention – in a good way. Books such as *Periods Gone Public, Period Queen, Period Power* and *Period Repair Manual* are popping up in bookshops. Companies that make period products are putting out ads that actually show blood and other period-y things as they are – no more blue liquid standing in for blood. Supermarket chains in Australia and New Zealand have swapped out the words 'feminine hygiene' for more straight-talking language like 'period care'. The managing director of Woolworths, Natalie Davis, says this 'a change we can make today that will help debunk the stigma of calling a period what it is and it will help many young women grow up feeling less shame or embarrassment.'[9]

Online, things are moving even faster with more and more social media accounts celebrating periods and talking about them – and other period-related health issues – in a real way. I love seeing this pushback against the negative view of periods and I'm all the way for normalising this very normal part of human life. Why should we feel ashamed and confused about something that happens to every human with female sex organs?

Another big reason I love this awareness and discussion of periods is that it's a great thing for endo and other health issues affecting the female reproductive system. The more aware people are of what a 'normal' period should feel like, the more likely they are to realise when something is 'abnormal'. One in ten women has endometriosis,[10] but given how hard endo is to diagnose and how normalised female pain is, the real numbers are likely to be way, way higher. Spreading the message that periods are something that can be discussed openly, and that monthly pain is not 'just part of being a woman' will hopefully mean that more women stop to question their own experience and think, *Hang on. Maybe this isn't just my period. Maybe I should look into this.*

When I was growing up, every woman in my family had terrible periods. For years, we thought nothing of it because we

---

9 7News.
10 Endometriosis Australia.

all experienced similar things. Turns out Nanna has endo, Mum and my two sisters have PCOS and I have both.

But even with abnormal pain or any of the symptoms mentioned above, there's ONLY one sure way to diagnose endo, and that's for a surgeon to collect specimens of tissue taken during a laparoscopy (keyhole surgery), which we'll talk through in Chapter 4, and send them for testing. But here's the issue: surgery is often considered a 'last resort'. Doctors aren't willing to request it unless they absolutely 'need' to. And because of this, most women will spend years suspecting they have endo; but until a surgeon confirms it, it's all a guessing game. This is why the average endometriosis diagnosis takes (are you ready for this) between seven and twelve years from the onset of symptoms to diagnosis. S.E.V.E.N. . . . T.W.E.L.V.E!

Can we let those numbers sink in for a minute. Think about the psychological impact of not knowing what's wrong with you for that many years, let alone the pain. Think of how much of a person's life goes by in that time. Seven to twelve years is just the average; for many others, a diagnosis can take even longer. I meet so many women who only learn they have endo once they run into problems conceiving after a decade or two of suffering through painful periods and the like.

In a weird way, I got lucky because my PCOS meant my endo was diagnosed earlier than it might otherwise have been. I was 16 and recovering from my second surgery – another cyst removal – when I heard the word 'endometriosis' for the first time. A nurse was talking me through the surgeon's post-op notes, in which she had mentioned seeing 'specks of what might be endometriosis' inside me. Instead of taking the opportunity to remove a sample and find out for sure, she simply did what she was there to do, nothing more. Endo was now on my radar, but I didn't have a clue what it was, or if I actually had it or not. Thankfully, during a procedure to deal with another cyst a few years later, that surgeon did take the initiative and, at 19, I got an official diagnosis. But others aren't as 'lucky'. This is why so many women with endo don't know they have it or how extensive it is. They might be in more pain than you can imagine, but without a 'justifiable need' to open them up, their questions go unanswered.

Adhesions (endo superglue)

One symptom of endo that can really make life miserable is adhesions. They look a lot like cobwebs, and they're caused by the inflammation and scarring that happens after surgery or after endometriosis bleeds. Basically, scar tissue forms in different areas and then adheres to each other. These adhesions acts as a superglue between organs that have no business being joined together. So, your bowels might stick to the wall of your abdomen, or your uterus might stick to a fallopian tube . . . again, endo follows zero rules.

As you can imagine (or may have experienced), having your insides stuck together makes life unbelievably painful, so dealing with these adhesions becomes medically necessary. Surgeons treat them by going in via keyhole surgery and doing what's called a laparoscopic division – where they cut and divide the lesions so they can 'unstick' your internal organs. I've had this procedure a few times. We'll talk through it when we cover surgeries in Chapter 4.

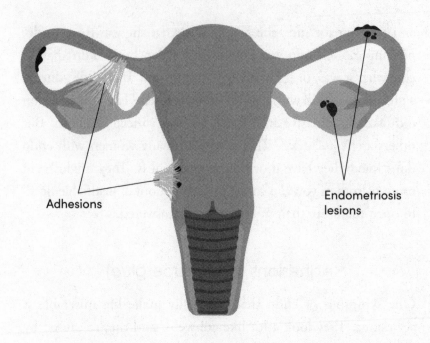

Adhesions

Endometriosis
lesions

This past year, I was in a TONNE of pain because one
of my ovaries was stuck to the side of my abdomen. During an
internal ultrasound, my doctor explained that during ovulation
our ovaries kind of bounce around inside us – apparently, it's
how they release the egg (how smart is nature!). They also
bounce around when we're aroused – I guess to hurry that egg
down the tubes so it can get fertilised. It's their 'We're gonna get
some' dance.

To help me understand, my doctor held my hip with one
hand while the ultrasound wand was inside me, and then he
gently tried to bounce my ovary. It didn't move. He said, 'See
how it's not bouncing? That's because your ovary is stuck to the
side of your abdomen. It wants to bounce but it can't, so you're
going to feel pain.'

For me, that particular pain felt like a deep ache – an intense pressure rather than a sharp, stabbing pain, but it's different for everyone and will also depend on which organs are stuck. As I write this very chapter, a section of my bowels is stuck to my abdominal wall thanks to my endo, and this causes insane, sharp pain when I've got a number two train moving through my bowels. It's the worst.

Actually, wait! There is one thing that's worse . . .

Clots happen

Clots – I'm talking big, messy blood clots – became a fairly regular thing in my life around the age of 21, and I've continued to have them on and off since then. If you're wondering where they come from, that's a great question. I'd love to know. If you find out, message me and share that info. Even after ultrasounds, the medical professionals have been baffled. They'll examine me and say, 'We don't know where these clots are coming from because you have no uterine lining.'

To which I reply, 'Well that's no good!'

Even though I may not be able to tell you where these clots come from or why they appear, I can tell you having a clot slide down your leg when you're minding your own business and living life is a shit experience. In fact, of all the symptoms that come with endo, I reckon clots are the one of the worst because there's no way of knowing when those fuckers are coming. There's no sharp pain to warn you, no sudden urge to go to the toilet; it just happens. BOOM! There it is, sitting by your shoe. I often feel the pain – a horrible pressure and ache – immediately afterwards, which feels extra unfair.

You may never experience this. I truly hope you don't. But I want to be honest about things that can occur and prepare you, so consider this your heads-up that clots can happen, they can be big (think golf-ball size) and they aren't pretty. I can literally pick my clots up, they're that solid. They feel like a ball of jelly.

If I'm lucky, I'll be in the shower when one makes an appearance; I'll be in the middle of washing my hair or whatever and then I'll look down and think, *Oh, wow! That's great.* If I'm unlucky, I'll be in a supermarket, or at work or filming a TV show in a remote location (yes, this has happened). Dealing with the aftermath of a clot in public is #awkward, but it can be done.

If clots become a thing in your life, I encourage you to accept that and plan for them. Please don't let the fear of having one stop you from living life or leaving your house. There are ways of working around them. Period undies might become a wardrobe staple, and you might want to stash a small endo emergency kit in your bag so you aren't left stranded if a clot strikes. I recommend stocking it with these basics:

- Undies and a pad (or a pair of period undies)
- Small pack of baby wipes
- Plain black leggings – they go with most outfits
- Small bin bag.

Then, if a clot goes down, you can shuffle off to the nearest toilet or quiet corner and sort yourself out. If you can, quickly pick that clot up and either flush it down the nearest toilet or chuck it away in a bin. Clean yourself with the wipes, pop on those fresh undies and leggings, bag up the dirty wipes/undies and either toss them or deal with them once you get home. Most of all, hold your head high and carry on with your day.

You might be reading this feeling horrified and thinking, *What if this happens in front of people? I won't be able to handle that.* But you know what, you will! I promise you. How do I know? Because it's happened to me – more than once. It flat out sucks, there's no getting around that, but you can't control bleeding or clots any more than you can control the weather. I used to feel so paranoid about them I wouldn't want to leave the house, but eventually my mindset shifted because I realised I couldn't be a hostage to this fear. I might have clots for another 20 years and I can't be a hermit all that time. I decided that all I can do is live my life, handle these unpredictable moments quickly and unapologetically when they happen and move on.

In my experience, people around you will be more traumatised *for* you than anything else. They'll be shocked that you have to go through something like this and they'll think you're such a badass for dealing with it so calmly. And they're right – you *are* a badass! None of this is your fault, and you have nothing to be ashamed of.

Treating endometriosis

Thanks to those 10 facts from Endometriosis Australia, you already know that there's no cure for endo (not YET at least – who knows what the future holds?). Most doctors will tell you that the majority of endo sufferers find that their symptoms settle once they go through menopause. The average age women in Australia, New Zealand, the UK and US go through menopause is 51.[11] Who the hell wants to wait until their fifties to feel better? Not me! So, let's look at the three treatment options. And yes, you already know I've tried them all.

1. Do nothing, see what happens.
2. Take hormone medications to manage the endo.
3. Have surgery to remove the endometriosis and/or resolve the effects of it.

Treatment option 1: Do nothing

Okay, I have to backtrack here because I lied: I actually *haven't* tried this option. It's not in my nature to do nothing. In fact, I think we can skip over this treatment since it's pretty self-explanatory. You cross your fingers, hope for the best and take a heap of Panadol and Nurofen as you wait for your symptoms to go away. I guess the plus side to this approach is that you won't have to deal with side effects from prescription medication or the hassle and recovery of surgery. There's a chance that this approach will work for you and things will improve, but in almost all cases, symptoms will stay the same or get worse. Do not recommend, but each to their own!

---

11 *Oxford Research Encyclopedia of Global Public Health*; The Royal Australian and New Zealand College of Obstetricians and Gynaecologists

Treatment option 2: Hormonal treatments

When your doctor suggests this approach, they're hoping that by regulating your ovulation and maybe even suppressing your periods, they'll be able to reduce the symptoms and slow the growth of your endo. I haven't had a period in five years, but it hasn't exactly been a holiday. I've had enough bleeding and period-like symptoms in those five years to last a lifetime.

Progesterone-like medications such as contraceptive pills, injections, implants (Implanon NXT or Jadelle) or IUDs (Intrauterine Devices such as Mirena) are often used to manage endo. But by far, the go-to hormonal treatment, especially in younger women, is the oral contraceptive, aka 'the pill', which is a combination of estrogen and progestogen. Sounds simple enough, but with over 30 different brands of pill on the market – each with a unique hormonal profile and their own list of side effects – it can take a lot of experimenting to find the right pill for you. And since each treatment takes a few months to 'settle in', this can be a long and un-fun process.

In 2020, along with all the other global issues there was also a worldwide shortage of Brevinor, which happened to be my birth-control pill at the time. I'd been pretty okay while taking it, so when I was told they'd just run out of it worldwide, my first thought was, *How does that even happen?* My second thought was, *What do I take now?* I was prescribed Norimin as a stand-in because there was only a 2 per cent difference in estrogen levels between that pill and Brevinor. I know 2 per cent may not sound like much, but when it comes to hormones, a tiny difference can create big changes in some people's bodies – mine included. I didn't adjust well to this new pill, though things have evened out over time. The whole experience just reminded me how delicate the balance is when it comes to hormones. We can't go chopping and changing hormonal medicines willy-nilly and think there won't be repercussions.

When it comes to the pill, I've taken Brenda 35-ED, Yasmin, YAZ, Brevinor, Norimin and Levlen, and I'm not even 30! I'm pretty much a hormonal guinea pig at this point. Some have been better than others at helping to manage my endo symptoms, but ultimately none of them has stopped my endo or even slowed its growth based on what my doctors and I can tell. That's not to say treating endo with hormones won't work for you, I'm just saying that it hasn't been the magic solution for me.

At the more extreme end of the hormonal treatment spectrum, you've got medications that induce temporary menopause. These are the 'big guns', and the thinking behind prescribing one of these is that by switching off your hormonal cycle you'll also switch off your endo. Logically, this makes sense, but as someone who has tried this – holy hell, experiencing early menopause is INTENSE. That story is coming up in Chapter 9 so sit tight for that.

Treatment option 3: Surgery

Not going to lie, I consider myself a surgery expert at this point. I've sampled from the endo surgery buffet and had a taste of almost everything on offer. That's why Chapters 4 and 5 are completely dedicated to navigating endo-related surgeries. I'm going to give you a full rundown of what to expect if a surgery is on the cards for you, as well as what to pack in your bag and how to make your recovery as easy as possible. By the time we're done, you'll know so much about these surgeries you'll be able to operate on yourself (jokes! Don't try that).

For now, let's just cover the basics. As you now know, keyhole surgery to get a sample for testing is the gold standard when it comes to getting an endo diagnosis, but it is usually a long time coming. Doctors will eventually (hopefully) say yes to performing this surgery if you either don't want to take any medications OR if the medications you've tried have not worked. While they're in there, your surgeon will probably 'treat' all the endometriosis they can see by either cutting it out by the root (this is called 'excising' it) or by burning it off (ablation). If there are any ovarian cysts, those will likely also be removed at this point as many ovarian cysts turn out to be endo cysts.

After that initial surgery to diagnose your endo, you may face more surgeries – especially if the endo they removed last time has bled and formed scars, creating adhesions that attach to other organs or parts of your body. Then they'll need to go in and 'unstick' those areas that are causing pain. Each time your surgeons go in, they should remove any endo they see.

If your endo symptoms persist despite these interventions – as they have in my case – you might need more extreme surgeries to remove the reproductive organs. Ovaries, fallopian tubes and the uterus may be removed as part of a partial or full hysterectomy. Thinking back to that list of endo facts, you'll remember that a hysterectomy does not 'cure' endo. Although some women (my nanna is one of them) swear that having the procedure has fixed their endo symptoms, plenty of other women will tell you that it has not improved their symptoms, and, in some cases, it's made them worse.

Any treatment you try is a gamble, no matter what you decide. Whether you opt to pop a birth-control pill, insert an IUD, have keyhole surgery or undergo a full-on hysterectomy, you'll find 1000 people who'll tell you that exact treatment was a miracle cure for them, and another 1000 who'll say it made things worse. Choosing is hard, but I believe that trying a treatment is better than doing nothing, and I'll roll the dice on that every day of the week.

What about complementary therapies?

This is an area I want to touch on briefly because although I'll be covering a few natural approaches to pain relief in Chapter 3, I know there are many people who want to go the natural route before they explore other treatments, and I totally respect that. There are plenty of non-invasive and non-medical approaches to treating endo, and if that's your bag, a quick online search will turn up naturopaths, dieticians, traditional Chinese medicine practitioners, massage therapists and acupuncturists in your area who treat endo and PCOS sufferers.

I've tried a few natural treatments in my time because I'm all about exploring my options. I've had a lymphatic massage (wasn't into it), plus I've seen a naturopath and taken gummies for better gut health (didn't do much). I've also tried the odd diet when I've spied a trend that's supposed to be good for endo or PCOS. Personally, I've found these approaches to be too much work for too little reward. I'm just not going to eat potato six days a week because it might cure my PCOS. My approach to treatments tends to be more along the lines of: *I've got six hours to spare. If I can't have a treatment that will help or heal in that timeframe, I'm on to the next thing.*

For that reason, I won't be exploring complementary therapies in this book. Not because those treatments aren't valid – I hear from lots of people who swear by natural approaches. I just don't have the personal experience or in-depth knowledge to talk about them here. But if you've got the time, resources and patience to stick with a natural approach that works for you, by all means, do your research and go for it! Anything that helps you is awesome.

PCOS

Polycystic ovary syndrome (PCOS) is an entirely different beast to endometriosis, but together, these two bad bitches have caused nothing but chaos in and around my reproductive system. Now that we've introduced endo, let's talk about the other piece of my health puzzle.

Like endo, the cause of PCOS is unknown, but experts agree that genetics and hormones play a role.[12] There's often a family link – your mother, aunt or sister may also have it.[13] This is definitely true in my case because, remember, Mum and both of my sisters also have PCOS.

PCOS gets its name from poly, which means 'many' in Latin; *poly* + *cystic* means 'many cysts'. The most common types of cysts are 'functional cysts'. These grow inside the ovary, and there are two different kinds: the first is a follicle cyst (these are the ones shown in the illustration over the page). These fluid-

---

12 Jean Hailes for Women's Health.
13 Ibid.

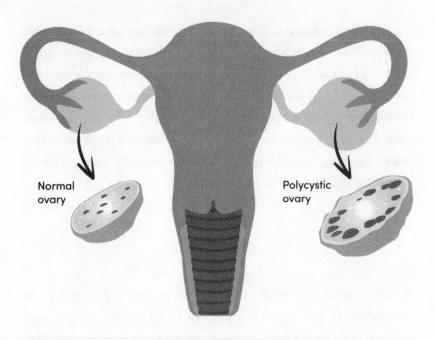

Normal ovary

Polycystic ovary

filled sacs are actually follicles that each contain an egg, but unlike healthy eggs, these ones never mature enough to trigger ovulation.

The second type of functional cyst is a corpus luteum cyst. It's caused when a follicle opens to release the egg inside, but then seals up and fills with fluid instead. Sometimes, these functional cysts go away on their own, but they can also keep growing until the ovary ends up so swollen and painful that the cyst needs to be surgically removed.

Different types of cysts

Believe it or not, some PCOS sufferers never develop cysts (they are in the minority) but most do. I happen to be a champion cyst grower. In fact, doctors have told me they can't believe how fast I can grow these suckers. It's like a game of 'whack-a-mole' in there; they remove one cyst and another pops up days later. Here are a few other types of cysts – and these ones can develop in or on top of the ovaries.

- Endometrioma – the blood-filled sacs we talked about on page 9 that are caused by endo.
- Dermoid cyst – cysts you are born with that are made up of skin, hair and nail tissues. These are solid rather than filled with fluid (we'll talk about these more on page 39).
- Cystademonmas – non-cancerous cysts that grow on the outside of the ovaries

My very first cyst was dermoid, but since then they've all been endometriomas inside the ovaries because that's just how my body rolls! (Like I said, champion cyst grower.)

How do you know if you have PCOS?

Talking about PCOS and raising awareness about it is really important because it affects SO many people – up to 21 per cent of women of reproductive age. That's a huge number, and the scary thing is around 70 per cent of people with PCOS don't even know they have it . . . yet.[14] If you're wondering if you're one of those undiagnosed 70 per cent, let's get into it!

---

14 *Australian Family Physician.*

There are three main symptoms of PCOS:

1. **Irregular periods** (for example, you might only have eight or nine periods a year rather than the standard 12, and they might be abnormally heavy)
2. **Cysts in ovaries**
3. **High levels of male hormones (androgens).**

Most of the time PCOS shows up just after puberty starts – in the teen years and early twenties – when those big hormones are kicking into action. My PCOS had textbook timing and my symptoms began shortly after my first period.

In my opinion, the high levels of androgens create some of the worst symptoms to deal with. Even though all females produce some levels of androgens, women with PCOS have higher levels of these male hormones, not to mention a shortage of progesterone, which is a really important female hormone that regulates menstruation. These out-of-whack hormones can create some not-so-fun symptoms.

Here are the classic PCOS symptoms to look out for:

- Excess facial and body hair (on your back, bum, thumbs, toes, face . . . anywhere really)
- Severe acne
- Male-pattern baldness (this type of hair loss often increases in mid-life)
- Weight gain often leading to obesity
- Fatigue
- Darkening of skin – patches of darker skin can appear under arms, on breasts or on the back of your neck
- Pelvic pain and heavy periods

- Headaches
- Infertility
- Mood changes
- Depression and anxiety (often caused by dealing with the other symptoms).

Again, just like endo, because many of these symptoms – pelvic pain, mood swings and fatigue, for example – get thrown into the bucket of 'being a woman', heaps of people with PCOS only learn they have it when they have issues getting pregnant and doctors start investigating.

This is why we gotta talk about it! The more familiar someone is with the signs and symptoms of PCOS, the better their chances of being diagnosed and finding treatments that work for them sooner. Early diagnosis is important for many reasons, but a huge reason is quality of life.

Living with the symptoms of PCOS can have a massive impact on a person's happiness, self-esteem and overall health. It's not rocket science; if you struggle with issues like obesity, excess body hair, headaches and pain for years, you're at greater risk of running into emotional and mental issues that become separate and serious challenges of their own. Tackling those symptoms earlier gives you a better chance of heading off bigger problems down the road.

Diagnosing and treating PCOS

Thankfully, PCOS is a *little* easier to diagnose than endo. There's no 'one test' that diagnoses it – instead, it's a jigsaw puzzle your doctor puts together, taking your symptoms, blood tests and pelvic exams or ultrasounds into account. Some PCOS sufferers will have every symptom while others may only have one or two, so it's important to keep track of anything you feel is unusual. If you've got a phone or watch with a period tracker on it, that's an easy way to keep track of your cycle and how regular it is, and what the monthly (or not so monthly) symptoms are.

Unlike endo, cysts caused by PCOS *can* be seen on an ultrasound, which is one positive because ultimately this makes the condition easier to diagnose and monitor. If your blood tests and symptoms aren't enough info to go on, your doctor might send you for an internal ultrasound (more about these on page 40). It's worth mentioning, though, that ultrasounds aren't an accurate way to diagnose PCOS if you're in your teens or early twenties because around 70 per cent of young women will display polycystic ovaries on an ultrasound.[15] It's a more effective tool once you're in your mid-twenties.

Confusingly, some women have PCO without the S. They have polycystic ovaries, but not the syndrome. This is usually discovered by chance when doctors are investigating something else. For example, an ultrasound might show lots of partially mature follicles in a woman's ovaries, but her health might be totally normal – she'll have no symptoms of PCOS, and no issues with her period, fertility or conceiving. It's only when you throw hormone imbalance and irregular periods into the mix that you have the syndrome.

---

15 Ibid.

Treating PCOS

There is no 'cure' for PCOS. Instead, doctors look to manage symptoms a few different ways. The most common treatment for PCOS is the birth control pill or some other form of hormonal contraception. The hormones balance out the androgens and provide the progesterone your body needs to start ovulating regularly.

Metformin, which is a medicine for diabetes, is another treatment that is often prescribed. It helps the body to process insulin, bringing blood sugar levels back within a normal range and hopefully reducing those male hormones enough that your periods become regular, and those hormonal symptoms stop being an issue.

A treatment option you can control and start at any time is following a healthy (or at least healthy-ish) lifestyle – we'll talk a lot more about this in Chapter 8. But basically, because PCOS is linked to inflammation in the body, diet can be one treatment option. I can't vouch for any PCOS-specific diets, but I've heard from women online who swear that their diet has helped them manage their symptoms. Either way, eating healthy food and getting exercise is never a bad idea, especially if you're dealing with a syndrome that causes weight gain and makes losing weight difficult.

Another treatment option is surgery to remove the cyst. This is done laparoscopically, and the exact technique will depend on what type of cyst you have and where it's growing – inside or on top of the ovary. If the surgeon needs to open the ovary to get at the cyst, it will be closed up using dissolvable stitches – or at least they should be dissolvable. Unfortunately, I had a surgeon use the wrong type of stitches once, and that was painful.

Finally, there's the treatment option that comes closest to a 'cure', and that's removing the ovaries completely. After all, you can't grow ovarian cysts if you don't have ovaries! This option is pretty radical: if you want to have biological children in the future you have to go through an egg retrieval process beforehand to make sure you have that option once the ovaries are removed. I'm currently pursuing ovary removal, but, as you'll find out, it's not exactly a simple process.

At this point, I think we're all agreed that PCOS is a bummer, and that it's very different to endo, but people often want to know if I think it's worse. My answer is . . . it depends. Some days, the pain from an ovarian cyst feels worse than any endo pain, but other days, endo pain wins hands down. Even though PCOS is manageable for the most part, it is still painful. The pain is mostly pressure related – a deep uncomfortable ache that gets worse as cysts grow. I can always tell when I have a cyst because I'll notice a familiar pressure when I sit up in a certain way.

My best advice is to listen to your body. If you feel an uncomfortable pressure during sex or notice pain in your abdomen that isn't going away, get it checked. Request blood tests to check your hormone levels, keep notes about any symptoms and ask for an ultrasound if you're of an age where that's an accurate indicator.

Sometimes, cysts burst

The thing about cysts is that they can burst, and I hardly have words to describe that kind of pain. When people ask me how to tell if an ovarian cyst is bursting, I tell them they'll just know.

Some people reckon it's worse than childbirth; I can't compare the two, but what I can say is that it's excruciating. Ideally, it won't ever happen to you but since I promised to give you the full picture in this book, here's how it went down for me the first time.

I was at home recovering from a surgery I'd had two days before to remove yet another ovarian cyst. I'd been in pain all day, but suddenly I was in agony – doubled over, unable to walk, passing out, that's how bad the pain was. I was scared and I didn't know what was happening, so I called the surgeon who'd operated on me. She told me that what I was experiencing was just post-operative pain and that I should take another one of the pain meds she'd prescribed.

I took another Endone, but I was very familiar with post-op pain by now and I knew this wasn't it, so I called her again, crying, and said, 'Something is wrong!' This time, she told me to go to the hospital and get checked out. My boyfriend, Mick, was away at the time but, thankfully, a friend of mine had stopped by. I dropped to the floor and screamed, 'Something's happening!' Yep. Something happened alright. A cyst had popped inside me, I was bleeding like crazy and the pain was next level. My poor friend was terrified as she bundled me into her car and drove me to the hospital.

No word of a lie, I entered that emergency department (where I'd worked on placement during my nursing training) screaming and shouting: 'You have to see me! I'm bleeding! I'm in pain.' Nothing about me was calm and collected; I was out of my mind with the pain. My friend rang my mum and said, 'You've got to come and help Erin. We're at the hospital and she's screaming at everyone.' Mum was there within minutes.

When the nurse asked what I'd taken for the pain, I told her: 'Four Endone.'

'FOUR?!'

'I'd take heroin at this point to stop this pain. Please give me something *now* because something bad has happened.'

'Ah, you've just had surgery. It could be an infection.'

'It's not an infection! Something has popped inside me.'

They set me up in a bed and a nurse asked me if I had any allergies because they were about to give me some morphine for the pain. I told them I would need an anti-nauseant beforehand, but that I was allergic to Maxolon (the anti-nauseant commonly given). As I watched the nurses from my bed, all I could think was that they were SO slow. I was full-on shaking with pain and getting angrier by the minute. Even Mum leaned over and said in Portuguese, 'These fucking nurses, they're so slow!' Because of my nursing placement, I knew things could move faster – I'd seen it with my own eyes. When the nurse finally got the cannula in and started injecting medication into me, I asked what drug it was. (This was her first fuck-up, by the way: nurses are trained to tell a patient what they are about to do and what medicine they are being given. This needs to be done *before* any medication is administered not during or after.)

'It's Maxolon.'

'MAXOLON!! I'm highly allergic to that, you idiot!'

By then, it was in my veins so I knew what was coming next: within a minute or two my jaw and body would start spasming uncontrollably. I started panicking and my mum turned to the nurse and said, 'She said that to you! It's listed as an allergy right there in her paperwork!'

At this point, a doctor walked in and calmly asked me how I'd reacted the last time I'd been given Maxolon – he was deciding whether or not I needed a drug to reverse the medicine.

I saved him the trouble and shouted, 'REVERSE THIS!'

They gave me a reversal drug followed by heaps of morphine and finally, I calmed down. But the next day, I went off my head at everyone. Imagine if I'd had an anaphylactic reaction? They'd been so slow to react, and it wasn't acceptable. After my next surgery, the surgeon told me that it looked as though my suspicions had been correct – a cyst had burst. Like I said, when it happens, you just know.

The next time I felt that type of pain, I was prepared. I took strong pain meds and got into a hot shower with Mick nearby. I got down on all fours when the pain got intense and when the cyst burst, all this blood just ran into the water and down the drain. This type of self-medicating probably isn't recommended, but I wasn't up for going to the hospital again now that I knew what was coming. If anything, it had made the last experience worse.

Every month, I run into at least a few women who have endo or PCOS and end up having conversations with them about their treatment. They tell me how they're on this pill for their PCOS or how they've been trying to have a baby for the past eight years while dealing with PCOS and I listen, I nod, I empathise, and – where I can – I try to help.

Just recently, a young woman told me that she's been taking a medication her doctor prescribed to treat her PCOS. Even though she's been on it for a while now, her pain is still so bad. Is that medication right for her? Maybe. Has her doctor sent her for an ultrasound to see how she's tracking inside? Nup. Has he told her that her pain is 'normal'? Yup.

Stories like this are so frustrating. I FEEL them on a deep level! By the end of that conversation, I was raging inside. I asked if she wanted me to call her doctor and ask about alternative medications, but she didn't want to unleash me on him (lucky for him). Instead, she said she was going to, 'leave it for a while and see if the pain improved'. I nodded and smiled – each to their own – but I walked away thinking, *Ah! Please let me help you.*

Never forget that doctors aren't these mighty beings with special powers. You *can* question them. You *can* push them to explore options if a treatment isn't working. You don't have to accept pain. I don't want you to bash your doctor's door down or anything dramatic, but I DO want you to be strong, informed and smart about getting the care you deserve.

2

xxx

How I became a
pregnant virgin

Let me paint you a little picture of me at 13: I was the baby of the family – the youngest of four, with an older brother and two older sisters. Even though I was young, I was already pretty rebellious maybe because I grew up watching my teenage siblings. I was into skipping school, talking to boys and doing my makeup – badly. (I'm talking mousse-foundation lines, over-straightened hair, heavy eyeshadow, the lot.)

I was desperate for my period to start (HAHA! The irony!) so I could be part of the same 'lady gang' as my mum and two older sisters. Periods tended to come early for the women in my family: Mum got hers at seven, and my older sisters both got theirs at 11, yet mine was MIA. Waiting for the real thing was so frustrating that I even tried to fake it, picking a scab and smearing the tiny speck of blood on a pad. I thought I was a genius, but when I showed Mum and my sisters, they weren't fooled for a second.

While I was waiting for my period, that awkward pre-teen phase hit me hard. I was chubby, partly down to hormones and partly down to eating badly when I was alone at home. We did have proper sit-down dinners together as a family, but Mum was single and working to provide for us, and my older siblings were in their late teens and early twenties by this point, so everyone was off living their own lives a lot of the time. My dad lived nearby, but he wasn't always in the picture while I was growing up because he spent a lot of time working out of state.

When I was feeling down about a few kids at school who'd started making comments about my weight, Mum took me to a dietician. I remember the moment that woman took my height and weight measurements like it was yesterday because it's replayed in my mind since then. She turned to Mum and said, 'At her height, she's classed as obese.'

Those words burned into my brain: *Oh, okay. I'm fat.* After running some tests, she told Mum that I had high cholesterol and sent us home with a new eating regime for me and a few factsheets. From that point on, the fridge and cupboards at home were stocked with my special spreads and the foods I had to eat to bring down my cholesterol.

Oh, and did I mention I was sort of hairy? Yep, I had facial hair. Actually, I had a lot of hair everywhere. Knowing what I know now, chubbiness, high cholesterol and excess hair are all classic signs of PCOS, but because I was so young and didn't have my period yet, it wasn't on our radar at all. Yes, Mum had ovarian cysts, and yes, both my sisters had classic signs of PCOS, but Mum is Portuguese, so a little extra sprinkling of hair isn't that out of the ordinary for women in our family.

One thing that was definitely weird, though, was my stomach. It stuck out so much whenever I lay down and was rock hard to the touch. It was big, but we all thought I just had a big tummy. There was also this pain in my stomach – not all the time, but it was definitely humming away in the background of my life.

Finally, at 14, my period made its grand entrance. I woke up for school and suddenly thought, *Geez, it's really wet down there.* Then, *Oh my God, have I peed myself?* Blurry eyed, I lifted up my doona and stared in horror. I pulled down the pants of my puppy-dog pyjamas to find my legs covered with blood. I sprinted to Mum's room screaming, 'I'm dying!' After looking me over for a second, she laughed and said, 'You're not dying, Erin. You've got your period.'

After helping me clean myself up, Mum showed me how to put a pad on properly, folding the wings around the sides of my underwear. Then, she started talking to me about how I should pack one or two in my backpack so I could change my pads throughout the day.

'I can't go to school!'

'You *have* to go to school, Erin. I've got to go to work. Sorry!'

'NO WAY! I can't go to school bleeding like this. We stay indoors when this happens, don't we?'

And that right there was my first lesson about periods: bleeding or not, the show must go on. Off to school I went. That whole day, I was paranoid that someone would clock the bulky pad I was wearing and think it was a diaper. Nobody noticed, of course. But I hated that feeling. And from that day on, my periods were terrible. Every month, the cramps and the pain would floor me, and Mum would say, 'You're so like your sister! It used to be just like this for her when she first got her period.' I thought, *Ugh. This must be normal.* It was so disappointing to have something I'd been waiting for for so long turn out to be this messy, annoying pain in the ass. I wanted out of this lady gang, but there was no going back.

Cyst number one

About four or five months after my period started, I walked into the TV room and lay down next to Mum. After a while, I lifted my shirt to show her my stomach, which was bulging on one side and rock hard. If my abdomen got that big now, I'd freak out and go to the hospital right away, but back then I just thought I had a fat tummy. I used to push it down and try to make it flatter, but it was super firm and felt so weird. I patted my belly and said, 'Look how fat I am.' Mum says she remembers seeing the bulge in my stomach and thinking, *What on Earth is that?* She had me at the doctor's before I could say 'boo'.

After examining my swollen stomach, the doctor said they suspected I was around 23 weeks pregnant. Mum looked at me, mouth open, with this *Are you kidding me?!* expression, and instantly I jumped into panic mode. It wasn't true! I begged her to believe me and insisted over and over that I wasn't pregnant. It didn't help that I'd started dating an older boy a couple of weeks earlier, but he was only my first boyfriend, and although I knew what sex was (sort of), I definitely wasn't having any.

Three urine tests later, the adults in the room finally accepted that I definitely wasn't pregnant. When two blood tests showed nothing suspicious, the doctor decided to send me for a scan, which revealed the reason for my swollen stomach: a very large dermoid cyst.

I know we've talked about cysts a little bit – so far, we've covered endometriomas cysts (those blood-filled sacs caused by endometriosis), ovarian cysts caused by PCOS and dermoid cysts which are congenital cysts – meaning you're born with them already inside or on you. Dermoid cysts often contain hair follicles, skin tissue, and glands that produce sweat and oil. The glands continue to produce those things, so as you grow, the cyst grows, too. Dermoid cysts are pretty common and can grow anywhere on the body. Mine happened to grow in my ovary. Because of its size, the docs were right onto it, and they said the next step, which needed to be done ASAP, was an internal ultrasound.

Mum wasn't going to be able to come with me to that appointment because it was last minute, and she had to work, but I didn't think that was a big deal. We lived right down the street from the hospital, so walking to the appointment alone was no trouble. Plus, it was just a regular ultrasound, right?

RECORD SCRATCH

We're going to hit pause on this story for a minute so we can talk about internal ultrasounds. If you've had one, great – you can skim through this section and remember how fun yours was, but if you haven't had this experience yet, pay close attention to these next couple of pages. I don't want you walking into your first internal ultrasound unprepared like I was. Trust me, going in blind will be a shock to your day *and* your vagina!

What to expect at an internal ultrasound

Say the word 'ultrasound' and your mind might jump to a movie scene of a pregnant woman lying down while someone slides that scanner thingy around her big belly. At least that's where my brain went. I skipped right over the word 'internal' – probably because I assumed it just meant that the machine would be *looking* at my insides, not actually *going* inside me.

Let's break down what happens at an internal ultrasound or, more specifically, a transvaginal ultrasound. You may be asked to get one of these early in pregnancy, or if your doctor wants to check for fibroids (a kind of tumour), polyps (a kind of growth) or ovarian cysts.

1. When you arrive for your appointment, you'll probably be asked to change into a hospital gown before you go into the room with the ultrasound machine. Otherwise, you might go into this room fully clothed. Then you will be asked to lie down on the bed. Your doctor might perform the ultrasound, but most of mine have been done by an ultrasound technician (aka sonographer). They'll come in, and have a quick chat, saying something like, 'Hi Erin, we're going to do an ultrasound to check out what's going on in your abdomen today. It won't take long.'

2. If you're still wearing clothes, they'll ask you to take off your pants and underwear and cover yourself with a sheet. Then they'll leave the room, give you a minute to

whip your pants and undies off, toss them on the chair
and then lie back down. Not long ago, I decided that I'd
had so many internal ultrasounds that I'd earned the right
to ask a few questions, so I asked the technician why they
bother leaving the room when they're just going to see
everything anyway. They explained that it was to make
the patient feel more comfortable and give them privacy.

(Next, I asked if I could take my socks off for the ultrasound
as well as my undies. They said, 'We prefer socks on.'
'Would it be weird if I took my socks off?
'Maybe a little.'
To me, socks felt like a strange place to draw the line. Like
having my vagina on show was fine, but bare feet were a
little *too* naked? I didn't get it. But hey, I'm asking the
questions we all want answers to!)

3. Once you're on the bed, the technician will knock then
   come back in. They'll turn off the lights in the room so
   they can see the screen properly, and they'll put on a pair
   of disposable gloves. Next, they'll ask you to bend your
   knees with your feet flat on the bed so your legs are
   up – the sheet or the gown will still be over you. Once
   you're in that position, they'll ask you to let your knees
   'fall open' so your legs spread apart. You know you're in
   the right position when you're feeling super awesome and
   not awkward in the slightest.

4. This is when the ultrasound 'probe' or 'wand' comes out.
   It's hard, cold, plastic and long – a little over 6 inches, to be

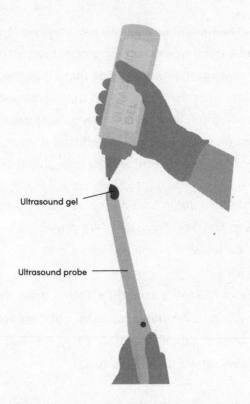

Ultrasound gel

Ultrasound probe

exact, though it's not very thick, thank God. It's attached to the ultrasound machine by a long cable. That thing, believe it or not, is about to go inside your vagina. Yep. It's how the 'internal' bit of 'internal ultrasound' happens.

5. Since this probe is used to scan multiple people a day, the technician will slip a sterile single-use plastic cover on it (a sort of condom for the probe). Next, they'll squeeze on a generous amount of ultrasound gel/lubricant to help it slip inside you easily. Occasionally, this gel might be warmed before you get there, but most of the time the gel, and the wand, will be cold as hell.

6. When it's time to insert the probe, the technician will do their best to make things feel as normal as possible, but there's nothing normal about this, so that's easier said than done. If you've got a sheet over your legs, the technician will lift it up so they can peek underneath and locate your vaginal opening. Sometimes, they try to be so discreet about looking that they don't lift the sheet enough, and I always feel like saying, 'Don't be shy, take a good look so you get it in the right spot first time!' Some women have told me that their technician asks them if they'd prefer to insert and hold the probe themselves – as it can be easier for you to guide something into your vagina than someone else. I've never had this, but I like the idea of having more control. If you think you'll feel more comfortable or relaxed, you can ask your technician if this is an option for you before things get underway. As long as you can follow their instructions and they can see what they need to on the screen, it shouldn't be an issue.

7. Once they find the opening to your vagina, they'll insert the probe slowly. At this point, they'll probably ask you to relax. Not easy to do when someone you just met is sliding a freezing cold 6-inch probe inside you! But it's great advice, so if you can, TRY to relax because it honestly will make things better for you. Close your eyes, if it helps, and take some slow, deep breaths. Try to notice if you are clenching any muscles in your bum or vagina. You probably will be – it's only natural. Tune into your body and let those muscles relax. Remind yourself that this is just 20 uncomfortable minutes out of your day. You'll be out of that room before you know it, so just keep breathing and think about what you're going to do after the appointment. In case you're wondering what's going on when the probe is inside you, here's a sneaky peek:

Transvaginal ultrasound

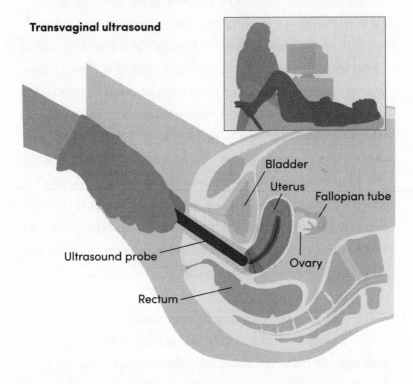

8. Annoyingly, once the probe is inside you, some technicians might try to make small talk to keep your mind off all the probing. If talking feels like a good distraction, chat away. If not, feel free to shut the convo down by saying, 'Sorry, I'm trying to focus on staying relaxed right now.'

9. The technician will move the probe around inside you during this ultrasound – slowly, but firmly, and from side to side. They'll push it against the wall of your vagina and make your insides move in ways they aren't used to moving, but they need to do this so they can see what's going on. It is uncomfortable, and if you have a cyst or adhesions, it can also be pretty painful. Again, try to keep the focus on staying relaxed and breathing through any pain. Remind yourself that this will be over soon. And if the pain gets to be too much, speak up so they can make adjustments.

10. Once they have the images they need, they'll pull the probe out slowly then pass you some tissues so you can wipe yourself off (the lubricant will feel sticky and yuck). After that, they'll leave the room so you can get dressed again. And then you're free to leave! Pat yourself on the back for getting through that and go treat yourself to something that makes you feel good.

I'm telling you all this and showing you these pictures to make sure that your experience with this is a walk in the park compared with mine. At 14, I had no concept that these types of devices even existed, so I would have loved a heads-up on some of the details. When the day of my appointment rolled around, I got dressed and walked over to the hospital. Mum was already at work, but she'd called ahead to give permission for the ultrasound and to pay for the appointment.

This clinic must have been in a new-ish area of the hospital because I still remember that it smelled of paint and had brand-new carpet. The technician who came to collect me from the waiting room was an older man. I can picture the outfit he was wearing. He took me into a large, cold room with an ultrasound machine, then sat me down to talk me through what was going to happen. That was when I saw the probe . . .

Now, bear in mind I hadn't ever put a tampon into my vagina, let alone anything close to the size of that probe. I didn't see how it was even going to be possible. When he asked me to get undressed and lie down, I remember thinking, *Shouldn't a woman be doing this*? But since Mum had organised everything, I just went along with it.

The fact that I still remember all this in so much detail makes me think that my brain is telling me, *No, you weren't okay with that experience*. The technician was kind, respectful and professional, so it wasn't nasty or creepy – but that didn't change how awkward and upsetting the experience was, or how my teenage body stored this away as a traumatic memory.

On top of the extreme discomfort of being half-naked in front of a stranger – an older man – and having a probe inside me, the procedure was also very painful because of the cyst. I kept my eyes fixed on the screen, where I could see the big white mass as the technician moved the probe around. That cyst was huge – and it was floating in a sac of bloody fluid. It was like two cysts for the price of one!

When he left the room so I could get dressed, I sat up, not knowing what to feel, and thought, *What the FUCK just happened?!* Later, when Mum got home from work, she asked how I'd gotten on.

'I didn't know they put it *inside* you,' I said.

'Oh, yes. I thought they'd explain that to you.'

'They did once I was there, but . . .'

It's not like I didn't have Mum's support, but with four kids and a job she couldn't be everywhere at once. In hindsight, I would have preferred it if someone had explained things to me before I was in the room with the probe in front of me or given me a choice between a male and a female technician. I think if I'd read about the procedure beforehand, then maybe I wouldn't have been so shaken by the experience.

If you want to bring a support person to your appointment – a parent, a sibling or your bestie, do it! Same goes if you think you'd prefer a female technician to examine you: ask when you make the appointment. That might mean your appointment needs to be rescheduled for when a female technician is available, but it absolutely can be done. Ask for whatever will make YOU feel more comfortable in that room. And always remember, if you're not comfortable and you don't want to go through with any type of exam, even if you're already on the table in the gown, you don't have to. You can walk away at any point – that is your right.

Another thing I want to reassure you of before we move on is that these ultrasounds will get easier. Just like a pelvic exam and a pap smear, you're never going to see this appointment in your calendar and think, *SWEET, I can't wait for that one!*, but you will breeze through them more easily. I've had that many internal ultrasounds now that I don't care if Mickey Mouse does it, I just want to get it over with so I can find out what's wrong.

You might walk around for the rest of the day feeling weird about the fact that a stranger has just copped an eyeful of your bits, but I promise you that doctor or technician will see another 20 vaginas and bums that day. Yours isn't special (no offence!). As soon as they leave that room, it becomes a distant memory. They'll remember your face, *not* your vagina.

Now, back to that cyst . . .

Cyst number one (continued)

Things moved quickly after that internal ultrasound showed the full size and scope of the cyst growing inside me. It was so big and I was so young that it booted the medical team into action. The doctor rang Mum later that day, referred me to a gynaecologist and told her to make an appointment right away. A day or two later, the gynaecologist we'd been referred to was talking us both through the surgery I needed, which we scheduled for later that week. Although he was explaining the process to both of us, he was doing that thing a lot of medical professionals did when I was a teenager: directing most of the conversation over my head to Mum.

At one point, he handed over a drawing of the female reproductive system, circled the area he'd be working on and explained how he'd be operating. I don't know how much of this information I took in. Probably not much. Everything was happening so fast that I found it hard to grasp it all. I barely understood how my reproductive system worked, let alone what was wrong with it.

Those weeks remain a blur, made even more blurry by the fact that my brother's wife at the time was due to give birth to their first baby any day – Mum's first grandchild. My cyst might have been the same size as a newborn baby, but there was no way it could compete with that level of excitement.

Operation day

As fate would have it, my oldest nephew was born on the same day as my surgery, and in the maternity ward of the same hospital. He arrived three hours before I went into the operating theatre and, I'm not even going to lie, I was really pissed off that he had to come into the world on my special day. That baby totally stole my thunder – something I still remind him of!

Technically, it wasn't my first-ever surgery; I'd had a few teeth removed the year before, so fasting before surgery and being in an operating theatre wasn't completely new to me. I felt pretty okay about everything the morning of my surgery even though Mum was freaking out because my sister-in-law had just gone into labour. Mainly, I was glad that this cyst was coming out – no more weird bulging stomach or pain.

But once I had the hospital gown on and was lying on the bed with a cannula[16] in my arm, things suddenly felt too real. The surgery horror stories I'd read on the internet a few days earlier (super-bad idea by the way – don't do this!) started creeping into my mind, and panic set in. I began crying and freaking out. The nurses around me did their best to calm me

---

16 A cannula is a thin tube that goes into one of your veins – usually in your hand or arm – before surgery. Once it's in, medicine or fluids can be administered through it as needed. You might have more than one.

down, but I hated the way they were talking to me like I was a little kid, saying, 'It's okay, Mum and Dad are also here and we're going to take care of you.'

It's not good for your body to go under anaesthetic when you're hyperventilating, so the doctors needed to calm me down before they could sedate me for the operation. They decided to bring my dad into the operating theatre to see if that would help. He got all gowned up and came in, but seeing my big, bearded dad in a hospital gown and mask made everything feel even scarier. Eventually, they injected me with Midazolam, and it worked like a charm. Within minutes, I went from full-blown hysterics to not being able to shed a single tear.

I woke up in the recovery ward feeling totally out of it. Someone updated me on how my nephew was doing, and then I fell asleep again. When I woke up from that sleep, I was alone because everyone was off visiting in the maternity ward (Hmmph!). I noticed that I was hooked up to a morphine drip for the pain, the type you self-administer by pushing a button.

The doctor who'd operated on me stopped by a little later while some of my family were visiting. He talked us through how he'd drained about 3 litres of fluid from the sac around the huge dermoid cyst before removing the cyst, which weighed in at nearly 3 kilograms (7 pounds). It sounded like a decent result. He had opened me up pretty much hip-to-hip to remove the cyst and then stitched me back together, so I had a long horizontal incision running just over my pubic bone – basically a C-section scar minus the baby. Years later, another surgeon would tell me that this cyst could have been removed via keyhole surgery but by then, the doctor who'd operated on me had already fled the country after being investigated for a cluster of infant deaths at the hospital while he was the head of obstetrics.

With my mum, dad and older brother still in the room, the doctor pulled the blanket back and proceeded to examine me. I was so out of it that I didn't say or do anything, but now my jaw drops at how inappropriate that was. I had no underwear on, and what fourteen-year-old in the history of the world has ever wanted their parents and older brother to see that?

The doctor told the nurses to re-dress my stitches, and then his hand must have brushed the tube of my catheter because suddenly I felt this pain inside me and started freaking out, asking what I'd just felt inside me.

Nobody had explained to me what a catheter was, let alone warned me I might wake up with one in. If you aren't familiar, urinary catheters are small tubes that go inside your urethra (that's the hole your wee comes out of) all the way up to your bladder. Once the tube is inside you, a tiny balloon attached to it is inflated to stop it from slipping out. There are different types of catheters, and different sizes of catheters and balloons depending on the age of the patient and how long a catheter is going to be used for (this will be relevant info in just a second, I promise). For some reason, this doctor had put a larger seven-day catheter inside me instead of the smaller 24-hour catheter, and because I was only 14 and had a small urethra and he had just knocked the tube, it was causing heaps of pain.

Urinary catheters aren't comfortable, but they are commonly used after many surgeries. The benefit is that, once it's in place, you don't need to get up to go to the toilet because your urine flows straight out of you into a bag hooked onto the side of your bed; you can recover without having to get in and out of bed. Here's a tip: if a surgeon doesn't mention a catheter when they're talking you through an upcoming surgery, I recommend asking if you're likely to wake up with one, how big it will be, how long it will stay in for and if you absolutely need to have one. Better to know what you're likely to wake up to.

Once the examination was over, Dad rushed over and pulled the blanket back over me. The rest of that day is fuzzy. Lots of sleeping and people coming and going between my room and the maternity ward to visit our newest family member. The baby was the only good thing about that day, but as unpleasant as that day was, the night was so much worse.

Catheter craziness

Mum wasn't allowed to stay overnight in the hospital with me, so she went back to our house. I fell asleep, and then at some point during the night – it must have been late – I was woken from a drugged sleep by two nurses. They were lifting the blanket that was covering me and one of them said, 'Okay darling, we're just going to take your catheter out.'

'I don't understand, what are you doing?' I said, half-asleep and trying to sit up.

'Just breathe, darling,' said one of the nurses, as she held me down. 'We're just going to remove it.'

Suddenly, I felt this sharp pain – I started crying and said over and over that I was in a lot of pain, but they must have thought I was being dramatic because they didn't stop. I'll never,

EVER forget how one of the nurses pushed me forcibly back down on the bed. I was sobbing as they pulled the tube out because the pain was beyond real. There was a good reason for that: the balloon holding in the catheter inside me had not deflated enough, so when those nurses pulled the catheter out, they'd also ripped the lining of my urethra. I started bleeding and blacked out from the pain.

When I came to, I was crying and crying, and the nurses were cleaning me up and telling me to calm down. They pushed my morphine button, and next thing I knew, it was morning. Mum was already sitting by my bed when a nurse came in to let her know that there had been a 'little problem in the night, but everything is alright'. She went on to explain that sometimes people bleed when catheters are removed.

I was lying there thinking, *No! It was not alright. I was pushed down!* I knew in my gut that what had happened was not okay but the nurse was talking over me so I kept quiet.

After the nurse left, I explained my side of the story to Mum, and although she was sympathetic, and believed me that it had been unpleasant and painful, having the nurse tell her first meant Mum assumed I was being dramatic about a common occurrence. She wasn't overly concerned, and I didn't know enough to push things further. I had to stay for another night, and once again, Mum wasn't allowed to stay.

Since I no longer had a catheter in, I had to walk to the bathroom to go to the toilet and to shower. The same nurse who held me down was on the night shift again, and she came in to help me shower. For obvious reasons, I was terrified of her, but I got up and went to the shower when she told me to. I still had two cannulas in: one for morphine and one for fluids. As she was undressing me, they got tangled up and she had to take them out. When she put them back in, she got them mixed up and put the tubes in the wrong cannulas. The fluids hit my vein so fast it popped up, and I passed out in the shower – totally naked. I woke up, still naked, with the nurse next to me explaining how she wasn't allowed to touch me until I woke up and could I tell her if I was hurt anywhere.

By this point, I was so distressed that I insisted they call my mum. Thankfully, the nurse finally listened to me and did what I asked. When Mum picked up the phone, I told her she had to take me home because the nurses were terrible. Mum rushed over to get me and, I think because of the incident in the shower, the hospital let me leave.

They organised my papers so we could leave quickly, and I suspect they probably didn't give us all the information we would have had if I'd been discharged normally. In the rush to help us leave quickly, no mention was made of how the anaesthetic from the surgery combined with the morphine I'd been on might cause constipation. Mum and I didn't know to look out for that or take precautionary measures. I went home, and after more than a week of struggling with pain that got worse and worse I ended up with a very swollen stomach. Back to the hospital we went.

This time, we went to emergency where a doctor felt my stomach, which was so sore because of the surgery, and diagnosed constipation. It was so bad that laxatives weren't going to cut it. I was going to need an enema. Once again, the what and the how of this procedure was not explained to me in any detail.

I went into that treatment with only the vaguest idea of what was going to happen. The nurse who administered the enema said, 'This will hurt near your bum a bit,' but I was expecting a cream or something . . . I wasn't expecting an actual tube to be inserted into my anus – heads-up, that's what happens! They get you to lie down on your side with your knees up, and then they stick a fairly large plastic tube right up your bum. Once it's in, they run a thick gel through the tube and into your bowels to loosen and flush out the hardened poo that's stuck in there. It feels so cold and weird having liquid pumped through you, and sometimes it's painful. But it definitely works!

Thankfully, the enema marked the end of the hospital phase of this surgery experience, and I was able to recover at home after that. But this surgery – the first of many to tackle things going on with my reproductive organs – completely scarred me, physically *and* emotionally. Because of the incident that night with the nurses, I no longer consent to having a catheter inserted when I have surgery. Most people don't know you can refuse this, but you have to consent to every aspect of your surgery. That said, I don't recommend that you refuse a catheter – it is often in your best interest to have one because then you won't need to get up and walk after invasive surgery. Without a catheter, you'll have to get someone to put a bedpan under you in bed and pee in that. As you can imagine, trying to wee into a bedpan while lying down after you've been cut open not only hurts, it also poses a hygiene risk. But because of what I've been through, I flat out refuse the alternative. If only someone had taken the time to explain catheters and I had been treated more gently, I wouldn't feel I had to refuse them now. Looking back, I wonder if they told my mum I'd have a catheter rather than tell me . . . it's possible. The phrase 'I'll let your mum know' gets used a lot when kids are in hospital, maybe too much. Knowledge is power.

I still think about those two nights regularly more than a decade later. It's one of the main reasons I wanted to study nursing – so I could make sure kids going through surgery never had to feel the pain, fear and helplessness I did. As part of my nursing placement a few years ago, I found myself on rotations in that same hospital, and lo and behold the same nurse who had held me down and mixed up the cannulas was still working there. She was older but there was no mistaking her. I had to let her know that what she had done to me had scarred me for life.

During one of my shifts, I stopped her in the hallway and told her that she was the reason I'd gone into nursing. I reminded her about what had happened that night, and how she'd held me down when I'd been crying and confused, how she'd refused to listen to me. She had the same old attitude, and brushed me off, saying, 'I don't remember that . . .' But I think she did remember, and I felt better for having confronted her about it. She might have a different take or perspective on her actions that night, but I know what really happened. I know the pain she caused and how she made me feel.

It was only after explaining all this to Mum as an adult that she understood what had happened to me. At the time, she had told me that the doctors and nurses had explained all these incidents to her, so I thought she had the full story. But when it came up many years later and I told her the details of my experience, she was in complete shock that I'd gone through all of that.

Be a 'nightmare patient'

Now, with another 14 surgeries under my belt, not to mention practical experience in nursing, I know exactly what my rights are as a patient. I know what the nurse or doctor is supposed to explain to me or ask permission for, and I make damn sure that those things happen. I go into every procedure, no matter how minor, with questions – a lot of them. If a cannula is going to be inserted into one of my veins, you best believe I want to know exactly which medicine or fluid will be injected into me and what it's for. If someone looks like they're about to touch me or adjust a machine or tube I'm attached to, I want to know what's happening before a fingertip so much as brushes me or the machine.

I go over the top when it comes to gathering information and I ask for what I'm entitled to – respectfully, but assertively. That might make me a nightmare patient for some doctors or nurses, but I don't care. I encourage you to be this type of patient, too. No matter how young you are, always remember that nobody is better than you and nobody has the right to touch you without your full consent. It doesn't matter if your parents are sitting right there saying everything is okay, if you aren't sure about something or if you feel uncomfortable, ask the medical professional what they're about to do and why. Ask them to explain it again and again until you fully understand.

Hospitals and clinics are busy places, and (despite my negative experiences) they are mostly full of good people who are trying to do the best they can with limited staff and resources. It's common for medical staff to be racing through the day on autopilot, so asking questions can be a good way to remind them to slow down, explain things clearly and fulfil their responsibility to ensure that you are as well-informed and comfortable as possible.

I realise that the stories you've just read in this chapter probably aren't filling you with confidence in nurses, doctors or hospitals, but I had to share them because they were a huge reason why I wanted to write this book. I refuse to feel powerless and scared like that again, and I don't want anyone else to feel that way, either. Hopefully, my stories will help you troubleshoot your own care – whatever that looks like. One thing's for sure, though, I don't want you to leave this chapter thinking you never want to walk into a hospital, so let me share these two positive changes since I had my first surgery.

1. Patient care has come a long way since I was a minor undergoing treatment for the first time. When I studied nursing a few years ago, there was a big emphasis on putting a human face on the patient. Instead of saying, 'Patient five needs morphine', we were trained to say the patient's name: 'Sarah, in bed five, needs more morphine.' Even little changes like this make the experience of caring for someone more personal and allow a more human connection.

2. None of the surgeries I had after this first one ever came close to that level of scary. It was the worst by far. So, it gets better from here, and by the time you get through the last chapter of this book, you'll be so royally prepped for any future surgeries that horror stories like mine won't ever be your reality.

Questions to ask before surgery

- What type of incision will you be making?
- What type of scar will that leave me with?
- If you have tattoos, like me, ask: Can you find an incision spot that won't mess with the tattoo?
- Will my parents/partner be able to stay overnight with me?
- If you see any signs of endometriosis while you're in there removing my cyst, will you take a sample to biopsy? If not, why not? Can we do anything to make sure this happens?

These are good starter questions. You'll find more on page 113.

The aftermath

Recovery from my first surgery was a pretty long road. Longer than I'd expected, anyway. I missed two weeks of high school and spent a lot of time in bed, on painkillers, sleeping, watching movies and doing heaps of homework to make sure I didn't fall too far behind. But schoolwork was definitely not my top priority. I was just trying to gradually get back to doing normal everyday things, like poo or sit up in bed. You don't realise how much you use your stomach muscles until they're suddenly out of commission. I developed a rash on my elbows from using them to push myself up off the bed all the time.

It felt so weird to be at home while all my friends were still going about their lives, and even when I went back to school, I still felt different from other people. None of my friends had gone through anything remotely similar, and they didn't understand what the surgery was for – it didn't help that I was barely able to explain it myself. To top it all off, there was also a fun little rumour going around school that I had been pregnant. In people's minds, it all added up: I had just started dating an older boy, my stomach had been big and bulgy, then suddenly I was off school for a couple of weeks 'recovering' with a long scar along my abdomen. So far, so suss.

There I was, about to turn 15, and the last thing I wanted was to seem different or stand out in any way. I tried to play it off like I was back to normal but there were still a lot of things I couldn't do because I was healing. I couldn't go running across the playground at lunch or follow along in gym class. It was a hard time. And things had changed forever – I was going to need check-ups about three times a year because of my polycystic ovaries.

Later, after I'd fully recovered, I became very aware of and embarrassed by my long scar. It wasn't a clean line – in fact, as time went on, I thought it looked worse. Whenever I'd go to the beach with friends and strip down to my bikini, I was so worried that people would see my scar and think that I'd had a baby – that they'd judge me. I was so self-conscious about it I'd use foundation to try to cover the scar before any situation where it might be seen. When it came up in conversation and I was able to set the record straight, the truth didn't sound much better – at least not to me. Sure, I could say, 'My scar's not from a baby. I had a large cyst removed,' but then a large cyst sounded kind of . . . eww. Now that I'm older, I'm all for owning your scars, and my advice would be that there's zero shame in them, so don't worry what other people think. But I know all too well that not caring about what people think is easier said than done – *especially* when you're a teen.

At the time my PCOS was diagnosed and explained to me, the doctor told me that any future cysts would probably grow on the outside of the ovaries, and they'd usually pop on their own. While giving my mum and me the run-down, he said something along the lines of, 'She won't even notice them most of the time.' So even though I was aware that I *might* need surgery when I was older, it definitely didn't sound like PCOS was going to be something that would have much of an impact on my life. I came out of this first experience with surgery and recovery thinking, *Wow, that was a big surgery for a fourteen-year-old. You did so well, Erin!*

But I didn't get long to bask in that achievement because within a year, another cyst had grown and I was back in hospital – this time for my first laparoscopic surgery. And then, not even two years after that, another cyst popped up so it was back to hospital for my third surgery. That first doctor had been dead wrong: I was only 17 and I WAS definitely noticing these cysts. I thought, *Shit! This is happening way too often. I didn't know it was going to be like this.*

Having my expectations flipped on their head like this was a shock, but there was an upside to it: I was becoming curious and starting to question things . . .

What else didn't I know?

What else hadn't I been told?

What might be hiding around the corner that I couldn't see coming?

Around this time, I stopped relying on doctors and nurses as my SOLE source of information when it came to my condition. I started looking around to try to fill in some of the blanks that clearly had been left. I also started searching for information and stories I could relate to from the patient's side. Since you're reading this book, I'm guessing you're at that stage, too. So, let's keep going. We've got a lot of blanks to fill in.

BONUS!!
Essential questions

Top endo questions from my Insta followers answered by Dr Tom Manley – obstetrician, gynaecologist and infertility specialist

How do you get diagnosed with PCOS?

PCOS (Polycystic Ovarian Syndrome) as opposed to PCO (Polycystic Ovaries) is diagnosed when you have two or more of the following symptoms:

- an irregular cycle (usually fewer periods not more)
- abnormal bloods (change in hormones in favour of male factor hormones)
- metabolic syndrome (hard-to-control weight gain)
- androgen side effects, for example abnormal hair growth or oily skin more prone to acne.

How do you get diagnosed with endometriosis?

Endometriosis is an inflammatory condition where cells similar to (but different from) endometrial cells grow outside the uterus. The most common symptoms are pelvic pain and/or heavy bleeding during periods, painful sex and infertility.

It can only be diagnosed with surgery and biopsy – usually laparoscopy.

Most endometriosis cannot be seen on ultrasound or other imaging such as MRI and CT scan.

What are the treatments for endometriosis?

Treatment of endometriosis can be broken up into four areas (there is no cure):

- diet and lifestyle – keeping fit and active and avoiding certain foods
- complementary medicine – naturopathy, Chinese medicine (herbs and acupuncture)
- hormonal suppression (contraceptive pills, IUDs like Mirena or Implanon, Zoladex) – all are aimed at suppressing endometriosis growth or reducing estrogen release from the ovaries
- surgery – should only be laparoscopy by a specialist. Excision is preferred when safe.

How does a drug like Zoladex help endometriosis?

Endometriosis is stimulated by the natural release of estrogen from the ovaries. Estrogen is released in response to the follicle stimulating hormone (FSH), which stimulates growth of an ovulation cyst on the ovary. Zoladex blocks the action of the hormone that signals release of FSH, which in turn switches off the ovaries and puts a woman into an artificial and temporary menopause state.

What surgical options are there for endometriosis?

Surgical options for endometriosis should always be laparoscopic. They would be excision or ablation (excision preferred) with diathermy or laser. Laser sounds fancy but is no better than diathermy.

Can you become pregnant with endometriosis or PCOS or both?

Most women with either of these conditions will fall pregnant naturally without need for treatment.

With PCOS, having regular periods, and therefore ovulation, is the aim. This might require some medication for ovulation induction such as Letrozole or Clomid.

Endometriosis might need to be removed surgically to increase chances of pregnancy.

Both of these conditions might require IVF if other treatments have failed.

Could a previous surgery be causing my pain and period problems?

Scar tissue or adhesions from previous surgery could certainly cause ongoing pain or period problems in some cases. We usually see this after multiple surgeries so it is important to minimise the number of surgeries to reduce this risk.

Why does sex hurt with endometriosis/PCOS?

PCOS is not usually associated with painful sex. Endometriosis can certainly cause painful sex, from either nodules behind the cervix, adenomyosis or general pelvic inflammation.

Are endometriosis and PCOS genetic? Will I pass it onto my daughters?

The cause of these conditions are not well understood but there certainly seems to be a genetic component. It is commonly seen in mothers and daughters or sisters.

What age is too young for surgery to see if you have endometriosis?

The most important thing is early diagnosis and treatment. Treatment in very young women (under 18) would usually be with the pill. If this suppresses symptoms, then surgery can be avoided or delayed until older age.

There is not an age that is too young but endometriosis will only occur after a few years of periods being established.

Why won't a hysterectomy cure endometriosis?

Hysterectomy does not include the ovaries, and estrogen from the ovaries is the driver for endometriosis. Even after a hysterectomy, endometriosis can grow back because of ongoing ovarian function.

Hysterectomy can be a good option for women with adenomyosis after they have finished their fertility.

Why won't some gynaecologists give the green light for a hysterectomy if the patient agrees to one?

Informed consent is the most important part of decision-making when deciding on irreversible surgery. When choosing a surgical option that removes a normally functioning organ, a gynaecologist may decide that removal might cause the patient more harm than good over a long period of time. When making a decision not to do surgery, the gynaecologist will always be trying to do the best by the patient.

How fast can endometriosis grow back?

The way endometriosis develops and grows is not the same for every patient so it is very hard to know how long it will take. On average, without other treatment, endometriosis may take one to two years to grow back. The amount of natural estrogen production seems to affect this, for example, the pill will suppress natural estrogen while a stimulated IVF cycle will increase natural estrogen. These treatments will have a dramatic effect on the rate at which endometriosis can grow back.

What pain relief do you suggest to help with severe endometriosis/PCOS flare-ups?

Treatment of endometriosis-related pain can be really difficult. Anti-inflammatory medications such as Nurofen, Naproxen or Voltaren help to block inflammatory factors released from endometriosis. This only treats the symptom though, and it would be far better to try and stop the pain by suppressing the endometriosis. PCOS alone does not usually cause pain.

What advice would you give to young people about endometriosis/PCOS from a gynaecologist's point of view?

I think one of the most important parts of treatment is to be listened to and taken seriously. The time before diagnosis is still way too long for lots of young women. When thinking about surgical treatment options, seeing a gynaecologist who is a specialist in laparoscopic surgery is also important. You can ask if they hold a position in a gynaecological endosurgery unit or if they are AGES (Australasian Gynaecological Endoscopy and Surgery) trained. This is the highest level of gynaecology surgery training offered in Australia and New Zealand.

Which areas of new research/new treatments into endo are you most excited about? And why?

There is some really exciting work being done in Melbourne looking at endometrial stem cell biology (Hudson Institute) and endometrial gene expression regulation (University of Melbourne). These are exciting because they might one day be able to directly alter endometriosis growth and ultimately find a cure for this terrible disease.

3

x x x

Make friends with pain (not really)

I'm sure you don't need me to tell you that life with endo usually means living with pain. It's the most common symptom of endo and it doesn't just come in one flavour: it runs from short, sharp stabbing pain to dull, throbbing aches. It can be a deep-in-your-body pain – the kind that a massage or changing the way you sit isn't going to help. You can feel it in your abdomen, hips, lower back, legs, bowels . . . anywhere your endo is growing. Some days it will be a quiet companion as you go about your life, other days it may be so bad you can't think straight, let alone get anything done.

Until scientists and doctors working in this field have more money to research the causes of endo pain and the ways to treat it effectively, it's on us to figure out how to live our lives well *in spite of* that pain. We can't wait around for life to begin; we have to learn how to work *with* our pain right now. Learning how to manage your pain will be the key to making the most of your good days and making the bad days as comfortable as they can be.

Over time, you might start to notice patterns; certain things may trigger flare-ups. You might learn that eating spicy food makes you cramp like hell the next day, or that you tend to bleed heavily if you've been pushing yourself too hard for too long. When you notice those connections, write them down in a journal or type them into your phone and then try to avoid the trigger as much as possible.

First things first, back yourself

If I told you how often people message me to complain that their doctor isn't taking their pain seriously, you would fall over. Details vary from message to message, but the gist is the same: *My doctor is telling me to take Panadol for pain that is way beyond that. What can I say to them?*

My reply? *Scream. Scream and yell. Make a scene. Shock them into taking you seriously. Hassle your GP/specialist/naturopath until you get the relief and the answers you need.* If the pain you're feeling isn't within the realms of what you know to be normal for you, trust that you know best. Nobody knows your body better than you do (duh!), and nobody gets to dismiss your worries just because they have a degree hanging on their wall. If you find this happening to you, please take action.

In my experience, it's mostly male doctors who don't get it. I've had too many encounters along these lines:

'Oh yes, Erin, that sounds like bad period pain.'

'Oh really? Is that how your period feels when you have it?'

'Well, no. I don't have a period, but I have two daughters, so I understand.'

'Having daughters is great, but that doesn't mean you under-stand what I'm going through, or that you feel what I feel.'

It's not right that so many people are told that what they're feeling is just bad period pain, or that it's normal and nothing to worry about. Studies prove that when men and women complain of pain, men are taken more seriously than women.[17] They are listened to more and treated more sympathetically. How annoying is that!

There may not be a cure for endometriosis (yet), but there are treatments that can improve our quality of life, so don't give up. This might mean going to different emergency departments and clinics, it might mean finding different gynaecologists and going to appointment after appointment until you are satisfied that you're getting the results you want. This searching might bring you good news or bad news about your health, but wouldn't you rather know you've exhausted every possible option?

By the time I met Dr Tom Manley in 2019, I was well and truly at the end of my rope. He'd been recommended to me by people on social media going through similar issues, and he sounded great, so I found his details and contacted him. My stomach looked like a pin cushion from my previous surgeries and my medical records read like a who's who of gynos in my

---

17 Harvard Health Publishing (Harvard Medical School).

city. I didn't have it in me to make small talk with doctors anymore. I walked into his office, sat down and summarised exactly what I'd been through, and also what I was looking for in a surgeon in the future. I was done playing games and I know I came on strong, but to his credit, he heard me out and really took in how 'over it' I was. Once I'd said my piece, he was like, 'Shit, okay.' Unlike the doctors I'd seen in the past, he was willing to consider my end goal: the removal of my remaining ovary so I could have a shot at living the rest of my life without cysts, surgeries and so much pain. He became an important person in my life for several years after that because I felt listened to, seen and – most importantly – BELIEVED.

The thing is, your pain isn't measurable, and that's hard for doctors. Ideally, your doctor will listen and help you find solutions that make your life better right now *and* in the future. But your doctor might also hit you with the old, 'take this anti-inflammatory', or 'try this herbal tea', and you'll be back in their clinic a week later in the same fucking boat. If you've seen the same doctor several times and made no progress on the pain front, it's okay to say, 'I know that this pain isn't normal for me. Please give me what I need to help with that now, and let's talk strategy for how we're going to treat it going forward.' You can also look for another doctor.

Natural painkillers

The best way of dealing with your pain is to find one or two non-medical painkillers that work for you and are easy to access whenever you need them. The two I'm highlighting here have seen me through all kinds of bad days, and I'm willing to bet they'll help you, too. But I also encourage you to spend time looking through comments and posts in endo groups online and asking other women about their go-to pain remedies. You never know what will work for you until you try it out. Some people swear by pelvic-floor physiotherapy, others are all about pelvic massage while others still love remedies like ginger tea or turmeric. Explore any that you think will help – there's no harm in trying!

1. **Heat**

    My number one, tried-and-tested, all-star, don't-leave-home-without-it method for pain-relief is heat, and I know a lot of endo sufferers are with me on this one. Heat relaxes muscles and eases cramping, which can go a long way to reducing pain.

    How you like your heat served is a matter of personal preference. Some want a hot bath or a hot water bottle. For me, it's an electric blanket, my trusty wheat bags and plug-in heat pad (bloody love that). I'm also a big fan of Hot Hands, air-activated, mini heat pads that stay hot for between 12 and 24 hours, which you can buy from most chemists. They are designed to be put in your boots or gloves during winter, but I love them because you can pop these babies under your clothes and nobody will notice. They are also great for air pain after surgery because it's usually up around the shoulder, and these sit right in the spots the pain tends to be worst. I'll talk more about air pain on page 98, it's something that can happen after surgery.

What I'm about to say probably isn't recommended, but I'm going to keep it real with you: I like my heat pack to be so hot that it's almost burning my skin. The hotter, the better in my book. But *almost burning* is the key – you don't want it so hot that it *actually* burns you. I just find it most effective when the heat on the surface of my skin acts as a distraction from the deep, internal pain.

2. **TENS machines**

TENS stands for transcutaneous electrical nerve stimulation; these machines are small battery-operated gadgets that work by sending mild electrical impulses to the nerves through wires connected to sticky pads called electrodes. You can stick these electrodes wherever you're feeling pain, and then electrical currents flow to these pads and into the body, interrupting the pain signals going from that area to the spinal cord and brain. This reduces pain, relaxes muscles and has the added benefit of stimulating your endorphins – your natural painkillers also known as your feel-good chemicals.

I was sceptical about how effective these machines would be, so imagine my surprise when they really did help with my pain. The relief I get after using one of these isn't to the point where I think, *Oh, I'm pain free!* It's more that I feel able to get up and do stuff. But to me, that's still a big win.

There are heaps of TENS machines on the market, and I've tried a few different brands now. All of them have been effective, though some have features I like more than others. I've tried brands where the electrodes have no wires, which is pretty convenient because you can stick those pads under your clothes and zap away without anyone noticing. I've worn this type of machine under my top at work and you really can't see it. Another good thing about a wireless set-up like this is that you can place the pads in two totally different areas on your body, which is great when you're experiencing pain in a few spots.

Another model I like has heaps of different modes and a remote control. You can adjust the strength and delivery of the electrical impulses in a few ways: for example, the impulses can be strong and come in waves or be gentle, and alternate from one electrode to the other. I really like having these different modes because pain isn't always the same – it can also come in waves. Whichever machine you go for, it will likely take some experimenting to find the right mode and strength for you.

As great as these machines are, don't get *too* excited. A TENS machine probably won't take your pain away 100 per cent, but, when used alongside a painkiller like Panadol, it can be an effective way of managing it. You could even keep one at home and another stashed in a drawer at work, then you won't be caught without pain relief.

As much as I've loved experimenting with the fancy TENS machines I've been sent because of my social media presence, I don't want you to think you have to go out and spend a shitload on one. You should be able to find a TENS machine on eBay that will do the job for $20. It might not have all the bells and whistles the others do, but it should still be effective. In fact, that would be a good place to start because what works for one person doesn't always work for another. It's best to start cheap and cheerful and, if you find that it really helps, you can always upgrade to a flash model down the track. Better yet, if you're seeing a physiotherapist or pain specialist, ask if they can loan or rent you a TENS machine first – or at least give you a session with one so you can feel it out.

Medicinal painkillers

My advice to people, and the advice I follow myself, is to sample a wide range of lighter painkillers and to try to get by on those as much as possible. If Panadol and Nurofen work for you, that's awesome! But if they don't help, speak up and get yourself stronger painkillers. Panadeine Forte (paracetamol and codeine) is my go-to, but I alternate between that and Mersyndol Forte, Endone and Tramadol, which are usually only prescribed for the days after a surgery. I cycle between these pain meds during my bad times because the body adapts to medications, so they'll stop being as effective after a while.

Strong pain meds like these will likely ease your pain, but they come with their own issues and risks: the biggest one is addiction. Endone in particular, which contains oxycodone, can be highly addictive. For that reason, you need a prescription for these meds, and doctors are cautious about prescribing them.

The more surgeries I've had, the more restrained I've become when taking these opioid painkillers. A while back, I wasn't feeling good in my mind or body, and I put a lot of that down to taking painkillers so often because I'd had so many surgeries, one after the other. I felt lethargic, low energy and just yuck. So, I decided to cut back on them as much as I could. If I woke up in the morning and felt I could tolerate the pain I was feeling or manage it with natural methods, I wouldn't take anything at all. I had days where friends told me I looked as though I was in pain, and that I should take something, but I'd refuse and see how long I could go without.

Often, I'd last a whole day without a painkiller and I'd just have one at night so I could sleep. For maybe a week or two, max, heat packs and TENS machines were enough to manage the pain, and I was happy that I wasn't on those pain meds. But inevitably, I'd need another surgery and wind up taking them again.

All I can say is: when it comes to pain meds, tread lightly. I'm all for taking them when you need to, but you don't want to rely on them for pain relief all the time. Strong pain meds are awesome when your body is rioting inside, but they can also make you feel out of it, anxious, tired and low energy. Over the longer term, that's not a nice way to exist, so finding that balance between medicine and other remedies is key.

After a surgery, take the meds that you've been prescribed, and then experiment with other pain relief like the options we've just covered. One thing that I often find helpful after surgery is moving my body, so try that if you're feeling up to it. Nothing crazy, just some gentle movement. I might go on level 2 on my treadmill just to walk. Over the past few years, I've developed a mentality of: *If I can do this one thing, I'll be fine.* It works for me.

Fight for relief when you need it

If your endo pain is severe, getting pain relief to match it might be challenging. You can even be made to feel like a druggo for asking for strong pain meds. I've been there. Five days before a surgery to remove a cyst, I was in fucking agony. I'd finished a prescription for Panadeine Forte but it was clear I was going to need a few more pills to see me through until surgery. My regular doctor was away on holiday (the nerve!) so I saw another doctor at the same practice. This doctor had access to all my records, but he flat-out refused to prescribe any more painkillers – even for just a couple of days. I begged him to help me, and explained that I'd been going to the other doctor for eight years, and that I'd had so many surgeries, and that my next one was only days away, but he still said no.

I was furious and out of my mind with pain. People like that doctor don't understand that by the time I come in asking for help, I am in unmanageable pain. I wasn't looking for a 'fix', I needed something to help get me to that surgery date. Instead, I had to white-knuckle it through four days of next-level pain with nothing but heat, TENS machines and Panadol, which is about as effective as a glass of water to me. When my doctor came back from her trip, she called me to apologise. I told her to never go on holiday again.

If you are in the early stages of your endo journey, pain meds can be a good way of gauging what *isn't* working. By the time you're filling your third prescription for pain meds, you should be like, 'Hey, GP, something is wrong here!' Ask them to refer you to a specialist or gyno who can help move things forward. If your doctor seems reluctant to give you pain meds because they wrote you a prescription the previous month, challenge them on that. Remind them that those pills were just to get you *through* the pain. They didn't fix the cause of it. If your doctor isn't doing anything to treat your underlying condition, what do they expect? You aren't suddenly going to stop needing pain relief if they haven't addressed the endometriosis.

Doctors, if you're reading this and you have a patient who comes to you again and again for pain meds, but you haven't referred them to a gynaecologist or other specialist yet, what are you doing? You are not allowed to make that person feel shitty for needing pain relief when you aren't helping them find a better solution.

6.5 billion dollars

That's how much money endo and chronic pelvic pain costs Australia every year: 6.5 BILLION DOLLARS! EVERY YEAR! And the financial burden on individual women with these conditions ranges from $16,970 to $20,898 a year according to one study.[18] I believe it. I've easily spent that much on endo in a year, not even counting the cost of unpaid leave.

Most of these costs come from lost productivity, i.e. the inability to work. And the main reason women with endo and pelvic pain aren't able to work? You guessed it: pain! Turns out the worse a woman's pain is, the greater the cost to productivity.

---

18 *PLOS ONE* (Public Library of Science).

This link between lower productivity and severe pain is also echoed in studies of European, British and American populations.[19] That means endo doesn't just cost the individual sufferer and their family; it costs the whole damn country. The experts who conducted this research had a good idea about how to lower the economic cost of endo. They recommended that 'priority be given to improving pain control in women with pelvic pain'. Um, yeah! Couldn't have said it better myself.

I've been very lucky when it comes to my working life; I have a degree of flexibility that a lot of people don't have. Not only did I train as a nurse, but around the same time I was doing my training, I wrapped filming on the reality dating show *Love Island*. When I got home, I started making money from social media, and this was when my endo pain ramped up big time and I ended up needing several emergency surgeries. During a year when I was in the worst pain of my life, I had a financial buffer that made it so much easier for me. This was the first time I remember thinking, *How the fuck do women hold a full-time job with this kind of pain? How do mums – especially single mums – cope with endo, work and kids?*

Setting my own schedule means it's easy for me to move things around for appointments, surgeries, or a particularly bad day. When I pick up shifts, I do it on a casual basis and swap shifts easily when I need to – there's no pressure to work a certain number of hours. Another bonus is that the people

---

19 Ibid.

I work with know what endo is, and how it can affect someone, which means I don't have to hide how I'm feeling.

Not too long ago, I had adhesions on my bowels, and it was horrible. I had picked up some shifts and was flat out at work every day. Although I was in a lot of pain, I didn't want to go back to an old mindset where I let pain stop me from doing a lot of things and living my life. Instead, I tried to do as much as I could, but it was hard! I wore Hot Hands under my clothes, which provided some pain relief. On some days, the pain was so bad I'd get close to popping a Panadeine Forte, but you can't take codeine or other strong pain meds at work.

One day, near the end of a shift, I could feel that I needed to poo (sorry if that's TMI, but . . . you know). As anyone who has ever had adhesions on their bowels will understand, the sensation of needing to poo is excruciating. It's not like being constipated; it's way worse. It's as if your insides are being torn apart because a portion of your bowels is stuck to another part of your body and there's no give in your bowels. They are rigid and don't move. It got to the point where I couldn't stand up. I was doubled over on the office floor, hunched by a desk. After asking a co-worker to cover for me, I crawled on my hands and knees to my manager's office to tell her I had to go. Luckily, I have a great manager who understands, and she was fine with that. The only thing was, I couldn't move. I was sweating and stuck to the spot with pain.

Eventually, whatever was in my bowels passed the spot where the adhesions were, and I was able to stand up and leave. I know how lucky I am to work a job that is flexible and understanding, but times like this make me think of all the people who aren't as lucky.

I've heard people argue the case for 'period leave', and I think that's a great idea. Sure, you can take sick leave, but that's only 10 days a year in most jobs, and, let's be honest, 10 days a year is a drop in the ocean for the average endo sufferer. But if you take more time off than that, you may risk being fired, or, at the very least, being made to feel as if you aren't doing a good job. Some employers also require a doctor's certificate when an employee takes more than two consecutive days off sick. This adds a whole other layer of admin and hassle, not to mention cost, when you aren't able to get out of the house for those two days, let alone drag yourself to a doctor's appointment.

Too many endo sufferers are stuck in workplaces that cause them stress, but they're afraid to quit because, if they do, they may not get a good reference since they've taken too many sick days. If they do get a new job, the cycle starts over again. Let's be real, who's going to sit in a job interview and say, 'Oh, by the way, I take time off every now and then because I have endometriosis, so I may not be able to work all the time.' Not likely! Instead, it's all: 'I'm such a hard worker and I have a great work ethic.' But that's such a shame because if people could find jobs that were willing to work with them, I bet they'd be more likely to be loyal to that company and work even harder.

Let's say, God forbid, you do lose your job or you aren't able to work for a while because of your endo, claiming benefits from the government isn't easy to do. Endo, like many other long-term conditions, isn't categorised as a disability in Australia, the UK,[20] the US[21] or New Zealand. If you meet very narrow and strict criteria that includes more than just an endometriosis diagnosis, it may be possible to claim disability benefits depending on your situation, but getting this help involves a lot of red tape and jumping through many hoops with no guaranteed outcome. As usual, nothing is simple.

Given all of this, it's easy to see why people push through their pain, doing whatever they can to get through the day. I get really sad when I hear about women who are in so much pain that they're either crying in a cubicle at work or fainting on their commute. It happens every day, and there has to be a better way.

Things seem to be improving in some workplaces: many companies offer more flexi-working or work-from-home options, and there is more of a focus on mental health and work/life balance, but overall progress is slow. If your endo pain makes it hard to manage your work life, my advice would be to look for a casual job that offers a lot of hours. That way, you have more options when making your schedule. Casual jobs may not offer sick leave or other benefits, but they often pay a higher rate. And remember, you're only missing out on 10 days of sick leave, which isn't that much, really. If you can find a job like this and push through the first four weeks, you'll be in a decent position to bargain with your new employer. From there, you're likely to be able to start dropping down the number of shifts and building a schedule that works around how you feel,

---

20 Endometriosis UK.
21 Centre for Endometriosis Care.

versus having a nine-to-five where you'll have a three-month probation period during which you'll need to be on your best behaviour, and after that you'll be locked into working the same hours week after week, regardless of how you feel.

A light on the horizon

For many with endo, managing pain got a little bit easier during the pandemic. Suddenly, they didn't have to wake up really early, get ready, drive kids to school, commute to their job and then put in eight hours of work before commuting home to care for kids, ageing parents or pets. Lockdowns force all of us to live life at a slower pace. We are free to take Zoom meetings in our trackies, have naps at lunchtime and stuff a hot water bottle down our pants whenever we are sore. And if a blood clot catches us off-guard, no biggie! A hot shower and change of clothes are just down the hall. That's a big mental load lifted, probably more than most people even realised they were carrying.

Many women have been reporting that their endo pain improved once all of those outside demands were removed – so much so that they felt better than they had in years and were more productive.[22]

Another pando positive is that more doctors have started taking Telehealth appointments so their patients can see them virtually rather than in-person. If this side of patient care sticks

---

22 Endometriosis Foundation of America.

around, we'll be able to get medication, doctors' certificates and all sorts of things without getting out of bed on our worst days. How good would that be?

It's a shame that it takes a global pandemic to prove that flexible working arrangements can be good for employees and businesses, but the past couple of years have taught us that a lot of workers with PCOS and endo feel much better when they have a working life that feels more balanced. Now we know this, we can't 'unknow' it. Endo sufferers have experienced better ways of working and now they're going to want to work from home during an endo flare-up or after they recover from surgery. They're going to want to take care of their health without compromising their productivity or income. They've learned that it doesn't have to be one or the other, and there are at least 6.5 billion reasons why a gentler, more flexible approach to work would be better for everyone.

4

xxx

Step up to the surgery buffet

I may not be a doctor, but I think of myself as an expert when it comes to the surgeries for PCOS and endo – from the patient side, that is. I've been around the surgery block and I've got the scars to prove it. This is one area where I can fill in a lot of blanks for you, and hopefully give you some insight into some of the surgeries you may face in the future. Since there's no certificate in 'getting surgeries' I can whip out of my back pocket to prove my expert status, check out the timeline on the next page – it's a little snapshot of my surgical journey so far.

I find it hard enough to keep track of all the operations I've had, so I thought putting them down like this would help give you an idea of how they've slotted into my life. You can fold down the corner of the next page over so you can flick back to if you get confused about what I have had done, and when. (To be honest, I'll probably snap a pic of this page on my phone so I can keep everything straight!)

Age 14

- Operation 1: Open surgery to remove a huge dermoid cyst from right ovary. No mention of endo.

Age 15

- No surgeries

Age 16

- Operation 2: Keyhole surgery to remove endometrioma (an endo cyst) on top of ovary. The doctor's notes mentioned that she'd seen what looked like endometriosis, but no sample was taken.
- Operation 3: Keyhole surgery to remove endometrioma in ovary. No sample of endometriosis taken.

Age 17

- Operation 4: Keyhole surgery to remove endometrioma in ovary. No sample of endometriosis taken.

Age 18

- Appeared on *Beauty and the Geek*
- No surgeries this year. (Yay!)

Age 19

- Operation 5: Keyhole surgery to remove endometrioma in ovary. Sample of endo taken and removal of endometriosis by ablation (burning). Finally diagnosed with endo!

Age 20

- Operation 6: Keyhole surgery to remove endometrioma in ovary. Removal of endometriosis by ablation.

Age 21

- Operation 7: Keyhole surgery to remove endometrioma in ovary. Removal of endometriosis by ablation.

Age 22

- No surgeries this year!

Age 23

- No surgeries this year, but my symptoms began ramping up big time.
- Appeared on *Love Island Australia*

Age 24

- Operation 8: Keyhole surgery to remove endometrioma in ovary. Removal of endometriosis by ablation.

- Operation 9: Keyhole surgery to remove endometrioma in ovary. Undissolved stitches in ovary from previous surgery removed. Removal of endometriosis by excision. Adhesions unstuck.
- Operation 10: Same as above (minus the undissolved stitches).
- Operation 11: Same as above.
- Operation 12: Same as above.
- Operation 13:[23] Unilateral oophorectomy (keyhole surgery to remove left ovary). Endo removed by excision. Adhesions unstuck.
- End of December 2019–end of Jan 2020 appeared on *I'm a Celebrity . . . Get Me Out of Here!*

---

23 This was my first surgery with Dr Tom Manley.

Age 25

- Operation 16: Keyhole surgery to remove endometrioma in ovary. Removal of endometriosis by excision. Adhesions unstuck.
- Operation 17: Same as above.

Age 26

- Operation 16: Left fallopian tube removed. Removal of endometriosis by excision. Adhesions unstuck.
- Next operation TBC: Unfortunately, it looks like I'll be having yet another surgery a month after finishing this book. Operation 17, here I come . . .

I reckon someone needs to give me a loyalty card like you get from coffee shops: *Buy five surgeries and get one free.* As you know from Chapter 2, my first surgery was a lot to take in, and it changed me in a lot of ways. Even though it was a terrible experience from start to finish, I'm actually grateful for that now. Setting the bar so low right from the get-go meant that the surgeries that came after were much easier because I was expecting the very worst. It helped me to become better at troubleshooting my own medical care and being an active participant in it; my confidence improved with every procedure I had. Now I always consider what can go wrong or how something might negatively affect me, only instead of feeling scared and powerless like I did that first time, I think, *How can I minimise that risk?* Then, most importantly, I speak up. That's what I want you to do, too.

The only reason doctors know that my endo is so aggressive is because my ovaries grow cysts like nobody's business. Surgeons have been operating on me regularly for years to deal with those cysts, and while they're doing that, they are able to observe and 'treat' any new patches of endo. They're killing two birds with one surgery – again and again.

I don't even want to think about how riddled with endo I'd be if I *didn't* have PCOS. In a weird way, I'm lucky because my PCOS has meant that my endo is undeniable. When surgeons operate on my ovarian cysts, they get to see, beyond a shadow of a doubt, exactly how aggressive my endo is. They observe with their own eyes how it can return with a vengeance just days or weeks after the last treatment. I've had doctors tell me they've never seen anything like it, and that they're shocked by it because it defies what they know from textbooks or research. I can't tell you how good it feels to be able to nod and say, 'See! I fucking told you it was bad!' It's evidence they can't deny, and validation that my pain IS real.

I'm all too aware that most women with endo don't get operated on as often as I do, and because of that, they don't get that same validation. All they can do is describe their pain, point to where it hurts and then leave the appointment wondering what's happening inside them, and whether their doctor even believes them. Not having your pain validated is one of the worst things about having endo. It's frustrating. It's depressing. It makes you want to scream at everyone. But mostly, it wears you down.

What are your options?

As I mentioned earlier, hormonal treatments are probably the first place a doctor will start if they suspect you have endo. Generally, doctors don't suggest surgery right off the bat to confirm endo because they want to avoid prescribing what they view as 'unnecessary' surgeries. Instead, they'll try you on different birth-control pills to see if one of those calms your symptoms. If you're lucky, one of them will. But if your pain and other symptoms continue at the same level, you'll be stuck having to manage that pain and grit your teeth through hellish periods month after month. After this goes on for a while (remember, the average time for a diagnosis is around seven years), you'll be dying to get some real answers and explore other solutions.

Pelvic surgery is rarely going to be at the top of a person's bucket list. It's not life-saving like an organ transplant, and it's not going to give you perky new boobs or a nice new nose like plastic surgery. The most exciting thing about the surgeries we're about to discuss is that they offer *hope*. Going into one of these operations, there's always a possibility you'll come out the other side with less pain, and that you'll be able to live a better life than the one you're living now. It's that glimmer of light – the prospect of some goddamn relief – that persuades so many of us to hop on the operating table. Again and again, and again. Sometimes we get some relief, sometimes we don't.

As I said at the start of this book, I'm not trying to promote anything other than advocating for yourself. I didn't write this chapter to persuade you to get an operation if you don't need or want one. Every operation carries very real risks, and that's why surgery – including surgery to diagnose endo – is often a last resort.

I understand the reluctance to put a patient through surgery, especially if that person is young, but how many kids get their tonsils out each year? That's one of the most common surgeries for children in the world, and Australian hospitals have higher rates of this surgery than the UK and New Zealand. Between 2017 and 2018, the hospital near my mum's house performed 394 tonsillectomies on kids 17 and under,[24] and a tonsillectomy carries just as many risks as a diagnostic laparoscopy. What's even crazier to me is that a recent study found that 88.3 per cent

---

24 Australian Commission on Safety and Quality in Health Care.

of the 18,281 kids in the UK who had tonsillectomies between 2005 and 2016 didn't even meet the medical criteria for that procedure and 'were unlikely to benefit from it'.[25] So let me get this straight: surgeons are willing to put children as young as two under anaesthetic for a surgery they may or may not benefit from, but when a young woman comes to them in pain, desperate for a diagnosis and can fully understand the risks of surgery, she's told no because surgery is 'too risky'? I'm sorry; to me, this argument doesn't hold up.

Instead of performing a minimally invasive surgery and giving her concrete answers, doctors will make this poor woman jump through hormonal hoops, often for years. They'll say, 'Try this tablet for six months.' And when that pill doesn't work, it's 'Try this different pill for a year.' I see so many women led down this path, and I've been on it myself for over a decade. In fact, I'm trying out a new pill right now. We take them like good little patients, and then we ride the hormonal ups and downs as best we can, trying to live our lives while experiencing side effects such as depression, anxiety, weight gain, fertility issues, blood clots, acne . . . the list goes on.

If you're lucky, you might stumble across a treatment that helps manage your symptoms; if you're unlucky, years will go by and you still won't have answers or relief. To me, it seems obvious that there are very real risks with this path, too.

---

25 *British Journal of General Practice.*

Looking back, I wish I'd had surgery with a good doctor at the start of my journey. Had a doctor taken a biopsy when endo was first suspected, I would have started from a solid place rather than playing a guessing game and having to muddle my way through years of medically induced hormonal ups and downs at a time when my body was still developing. A similar guessing game plays out for many sufferers because diagnostic surgery seems to be plan Y or Z, rather than plan A or B.

You will probably struggle to find a surgeon who will agree to perform the surgery you want – whatever that is. They'll try to steer you towards non-surgical treatments but ultimately, you should be allowed to chart your own course. This is your life, not theirs. Don't be afraid to draw a line in the sand and say, 'Can I have a diagnosis now, please? No more of this "I think, I think, I think . . ." It's time to go in there to see what the situation is.'

With that in mind, let me give you an overview of the surgeries you're likely to find on the endo and PCOS treatment menus. Let's start with the gold standard in pelvic surgery: laparoscopic surgery.

Laparoscopic surgery: gateway to the pelvis

Also known as 'keyhole surgery', 'minimally invasive surgery' (MIS) or 'band-aid surgery', laparoscopic is the least invasive type of surgery because it's done via incisions that are so small you won't need stitches afterwards, just band aids. Because of

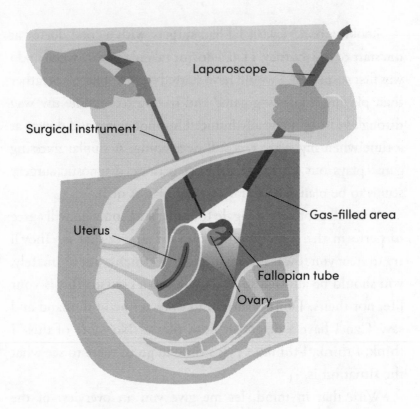

Laparoscope

Surgical instrument

Gas-filled area

Uterus

Fallopian tube

Ovary

that, there's minimal bleeding, low risk of infection, less scarring, less pain and less recovery time than with other surgery. Most surgical treatments for endo and PCOS are performed by laparoscopy, so it's a great place for us to start.

Keyhole surgery is usually performed under general anaesthetic. A nurse inserts a cannula into a vein in your arm and, once you're wheeled into the operating theatre, the anaesthetist (the person in charge of putting you to sleep and keeping you that way until the operation is over) administers the medication. You'll be out like a light within two minutes and you won't feel or hear a thing.

The surgeon makes one or more small incisions in your abdomen, usually in the belly button, then they insert a tiny fibre-optic cable with a camera attached to the end (a laparoscope) into one of the holes so they can see inside your abdomen. Images from that camera are projected onto a screen in the operating theatre so the surgeon can see everything. Another tube will be inserted into your abdomen to pump gas into the abdominal cavity – blowing it up like this gives the surgeon more room to move the camera and surgical tools around – and the tools will be inserted into another hole near the area they're operating on. How many incisions you need will depend on which type of surgery you're having and the goal of that particular laparoscopy. You can ask about the incisions when you book in for surgery.

The surgeon will move the camera to find out what's going on with your uterus, ovaries, fallopian tubes, bowel, bladder . . . the whole lot. They will also manipulate the surgical tools from outside your body and perform the surgery in a precise way. Opposite is a side view to give you an idea of how this surgery works. It's actually pretty cool.

All of the surgeries I've had, with the exception of that first one, have been keyhole surgeries. I'd been expecting a keyhole surgery the first time but, as you know, I woke up to find I'd had an 'open surgery'. That was a shock, but if an ovarian cyst is unusually large (like mine was) or not filled with fluid (which mine wasn't) then a larger hole is needed to extract it. Open surgery might be necessary if there are complications during a keyhole surgery, though this isn't common. If you're scheduled to have a laparoscopy, it's worth asking your surgeon if there's a chance you'll need an open surgery. This isn't to make you anxious, it's just so you can get your head around that possibility. The recovery from that type of surgery is quite different, so it's not the sort of thing you want to wake up and be surprised by, like I was.

AIR PAIN

Speaking of surprises, one of the biggest shocks I got when recovering from my first laparoscopic surgery was how FREAKIN' painful air bubbles are. They sound cute but they are evil little bastards. Here's how you get them: after the operation, the surgeon will press on your abdomen to push out the gas they pumped into you via the open keyhole/s. But there's no guarantee that all the gas will get out. It's really common for some of that gas to get pushed to another part of your body. Since it's not meant to be there, the bubbles cause pain. This air pain is also called 'shoulder-tip pain', which makes sense because the pain definitely tends to be up around my shoulders or ribs. If you have air pain, all you can do is wait for those bubbles to dissolve into your body. And you're not going to like hearing this but it can take anywhere from three days to two weeks for the pain to stop.

Apparently, walking is the best remedy for air pain, but I can't say for sure because in my experience, walking is often not possible – it's too bloody painful – so I always tell people not to feel bad if they can't walk it off. When I have air pain, all I can do is lie perfectly still. Most of the time I can only take short, shallow breaths because it hurts that badly – way worse than the incisions. It's a sharp pain and it totally sucks.

I wish I could say I've got some magic trick for you, but I don't. Time, painkillers, some distracting TV and lying very still are the best options for me. Also, as I've said, heat helps – specifically wheat packs. I put heat on top of the air bubble constantly because the burning sensation distracts me from the pain. Air pain is not fun, but at least now if it happens, you'll be prepared for it and you'll know that it's totally normal and, most importantly, that it will stop eventually.

Apparently, there are at least 11 strategies surgeons can use to try to decrease the chances of you experiencing this air pain, including using an alternative gas to CO_2 or using warmed or warmed and humidified CO_2. I suggest asking your surgeon how they're going to minimise the risk of air pain in your surgery. If they aren't sure, share this research with them (full link at the back of this book).[26]

---

26 *Journal of the Chinese Medical Association.*

The following treatments are the most common surgeries prescribed for PCOS and endo sufferers, and they're usually performed via keyhole surgery.

Ablation: This is when endo lesions are burned away by laser or high-frequency electric currents (diathermy). I don't rate ablation because the endo is not being removed completely – the top layer is just being burned away. The roots of the lesions are still embedded in your body; they're hanging out under that charred surface waiting to spring back into action. To me, burning is a temporary solution to a bigger problem, but even so, it's still one of the most common endo treatments because most gynos are able to do it themselves, and that makes it easier for the patient to get and cheaper to pay for.

Excision: This is when endometriosis lesions are 'excised' or cut out from wherever they are growing, roots and all. A scalpel or laser is used, and the endo that's removed is either destroyed (yesss! Destroy it!) or sent for a biopsy if the patient hasn't been officially diagnosed yet. Excision is considered the best treatment for endo because it completely removes it. Symptoms are often reduced after surgery, so you may feel better for a while or for a long time. If you're super lucky, your endo might not come back – but don't get too excited, I said *might*. Mine comes back almost immediately. Endo follows no rules, remember? This operation needs to be done by a gyno who is an excision specialist – it's a more precise operation than ablation and requires more training. This also makes it a bit more expensive.

NEW INFORMATION ALERT!

Ablation and excision are the most common treatments for endo. But, in the process of writing this book, I've learned that researchers in the UK believe there's a good chance that these treatments may not be all they're cracked up to be. Not only do they not improve symptoms or relieve pain a lot of the time, but they might even be making endo symptoms worse for a lot of sufferers (EXCUSE ME, UNIVERSE!!!).[27] If you're like me and you've had several of these treatments already, you probably find this information hard to swallow. This is exactly why we need more research to find better ways to diagnose and treat this common condition ASAP!

Remember those three types of endo we talked about in Chapter 1? Well, 80 per cent of endo patients have the first type: superficial peritoneal endometriosis. With this type, pain isn't necessarily caused by the endo itself, but by the way that the endo interacts with the nerves in the pelvis.

And here's where the new research comes in: it seems that a lot of patients with this first type of endo also have 'high degrees of neuropathic pain' – which is pain caused by damaged nerve endings. The research

27 *The Guardian.*

team at Oxford University believes nerve damage develops in three ways in endo patients:

1. The nerves around endo lesions get super sensitive.
2. Endo lesions push on the nerves and cause pain.
3. Nerves get damaged when the endo is treated surgically.

Nerves and blood cells can grow *inside* endo lesions, so when surgeons slice through those to remove the lesion it can end up causing *more* neuropathic pain, not less.

The research doesn't say that burning and excision *definitely* causes more pain, but it suggests there is a link, and that doctors need to pay more attention to the type of endo a patient has before prescribing surgery. They're talking about a move away from a 'one size fits all' approach to treating endo.

This research stopped me in my tracks because my endo pain only got worse when I turned 19 and had a sample of endo removed for a biopsy. That endo was then treated and, all of a sudden, my body went BANG! Was that because I have the type of endo that doesn't respond to surgery? Or was it because I was taking different hormone pills at the time to try to reduce my cysts? I don't know the answer; I'm just sitting here with you, looking at this information, and wondering whether these surgeries, which I've had so many times, are helping or harming me.

I'm not saying go and cancel your upcoming surgery or swear off surgeons forever, but it's worth discussing this research with your doctor. I'm going to. I think it's also a good reminder for all of us to have a quick google every few months to see if any new stories about endo research or treatments are being talked about. If you come across something you're curious about, send that info to your doctor or surgeon. Talk about it with them. If someone is on the frontlines treating endo, they should be across the latest science and happy to talk about it. That's literally their job!

Ovarian cyst removal: How an ovarian cyst (or cysts) is removed will depend on where it's located and what type of cyst it is. If it's on top of an ovary, the surgeon will either drain the fluid from the cyst or remove it entirely by cutting it out. If a cyst is located *inside* the ovary, then the surgeon will create a wedge-shaped flap in the ovary itself, remove the cyst, and then stitch the ovary back up. Once the cyst is drained (or if it's small enough), they'll pull it out through one of the little keyholes and toss it in the bin where it belongs.

Adhesiolysis: Remember those adhesions we talked about in Chapter 1? They're caused when scar tissue – usually created by past surgeries – sticks to organs or other scar tissue. They look like thick cobwebs holding bits of your insides together. Well, this surgery 'unsticks' whatever is stuck and cuts out those adhesions. Since adhesions don't show up on scans, you'll only have this type of surgery if your adhesions have been causing you enough pain and discomfort that your doctor has agreed to go in to look for them *or* if your surgeon happens to spot them while they're operating on you for something else.

Because surgery causes most adhesions, there's a chance that they'll either return or that this latest surgery will create new ones. If adhesions are affecting your bowels, then you might need a specialist bowel surgeon to perform a separate surgery to ensure those adhesions are removed without causing further issues.

Oophorectomy: (What a name, right!) This is the complete removal of the ovaries. If only one ovary is removed, then it's called an 'unilateral oophorectomy' (that's what I've had, though I am living for the day when they'll take the other one). There are several reasons for removing an ovary: a patient might have ovarian cancer or be predisposed to ovarian cancer; their ovary might be twisted; there may an abscess in the ovary and fallopian tube; their endometriosis might be so severe (it me!) that this is a way to lessen those symptoms; that ovary happens to be a cyst-producing machine – like mine.

Removing your body's estrogen factories can settle endo, since it's triggered by hormones. And ovary removal is also a guaranteed way to resolve PCOS – you can't grow ovarian cysts with no ovaries. However, since ovaries are also egg-making factories, doctors are VERY reluctant to remove them in people who are of child-bearing age. Too reluctant, if you ask me.

Removing both ovaries means no more eggs *and* no more estrogen, so this surgery sends the body into what's known as 'surgical menopause' meaning you'll be permanently reliant on hormone replacement therapy to make up for the missing estrogen. Taking hormones long-term carries its own set of risks (stroke, heart attack, etc.), which is another reason why this surgery is viewed as an absolute last resort.

Most of the time, ovary removal will be done by keyhole surgery. The surgeon will detach the ovary from the surrounding tissue and blood supply before removing it through one of the tiny keyholes. But it can also be done by 'laparotomy', which is an 'open' surgery where a long incision is made in the abdomen. Again, you have to ask a lot of questions before surgery so you know exactly how yours will be performed, and whether an open surgery might be on the cards.

Hysterectomy: When it comes to treating endo, this is the biggest treatment on offer – the nuclear option. This operation can either be 'total' (removal of the uterus and cervix); 'partial' (uterus only); or what I like to call 'the whole shebang': a hysterectomy and salpingo-oophorectomy, which means uterus, cervix, ovaries *and* fallopian tubes. A hysterectomy will put an end to your period, as well as heavy and abnormal bleeding, and can also relieve the symptoms of endometriosis.

This is pretty much the end of the road when it comes to surgical treatments. Not only is it a big surgery with a fairly long recovery time, the results are permanent. Without a uterus, your option to carry a child is gone. And if ovary removal is also part of this surgery plan, it is worth looking into freezing some eggs beforehand (if you want kids, of course).

Having a hysterectomy will send you into surgical menopause, and for all of these reasons (but mostly the baby thing), doctors will only approve this surgery if they feel every other option has been exhausted. Getting to that point – let me assure you – is exhausting in itself.

There are three ways this surgery might be performed, and it's pretty much definite you'll be put under general anaesthetic.

1. Abdominal hysterectomy: the uterus is removed via an incision in the lower abdomen

2. Vaginal hysterectomy: an incision is made in the top of the vaginal canal, and the uterus is removed via that incision

3. Laparoscopically assisted vaginal hysterectomy (LAVH): keyhole surgery allows for the camera and surgical tools to be used, and the uterus is removed via an incision at the top of the vagina

As you already know from the 10 endo facts, there's no guarantee a hysterectomy will resolve endometriosis symptoms – especially if the ovaries are not removed at the same time.

Removing the uterus and cervix ends periods but, as we know, endo can grow anywhere, and if the ovaries are still firing away, the estrogen they produce can still trigger endo to bleed month after month.

The same day my nanna gave birth to my dad (her only child), her doctor removed her uterus, cervix and ovaries because her endometriosis was so bad and he felt this was the best treatment option for her. He had no issues performing this surgery because, by having a child, she'd fulfilled her 'womanly duties' – at least in the eyes of 1960s society. When Nanna and I talk about my pain or symptoms, she'll often ask me why I don't have a hysterectomy. I have to remind her that it's because I haven't popped out a kid yet so the doctors don't want to do it. If I had, I'm sure it would be a different story. When it comes to women's health, I feel like the medical world is still stuck in that 1960s mindset, with those same old-fashioned views about what it means to be a woman. (I have a lot to say about this; it's in Chapter 9 if you want to skip ahead.)

Nan reckons having a hysterectomy did wonders for her, and she's had a pain-free life ever since, but go on any endo forum and you'll find many women who say the opposite. The science is inconclusive, so all we have to guide us are the experiences of those who've gone before us. What you decide to do with your body comes down to what feels right for you, what a trusted doctor is saying, and what the research you've done is telling you. Like any endo treatment, it's a roll of the dice.

Now that we've covered the usual surgery suspects, let's cover two other procedures you may come across, especially if heavy bleeding is an issue for you like it has been for me.

Endometrial ablation: This procedure sounds similar to the ablation we talked about before, but it's very different. For one thing, it's not a keyhole surgery; it's done via the vagina. The ablation tool is inserted into the vaginal canal and up into the uterus. Often, the surgeon will pop a tiny camera on a wire up into the uterus before this step so they can get a good look around the uterus and work out which areas they're going to target.

In this procedure, the lining of the uterus (the endometrium) is the target, not the endo lesions. Remember, endo tissue grows *outside* the uterus, not inside it. And though it's *similar* to endometrial tissue, it's NOT the same. Your doctor might suggest this procedure if your periods are very heavy and you aren't planning to have children in the future. The goal here is to reduce heavy menstrual bleeding. It will not improve your endo pain.

Dilation and curettage (D&C): A bit like endometrial ablation, a D&C might be done if you have heavy bleeding and your doctor needs to investigate or diagnose what the hell is going on in your uterus. In this procedure, the vagina and cervix are cleaned out with an antibacterial scrub before a special instrument is used to hold the top of the cervix still. Then the cervix is slowly 'dilated' to open it up more – either using medication or small dilators. Next, a sharp metal spoon-shaped instrument called a 'curette' is inserted into the uterus and used to gently scrape the lining (the endometrium), either to remove anything unusual on the lining such as polyps, scar tissue or any unusual growths, or to collect a sample of the lining to be sent for testing. Sometimes, instead of mostly using a curette, the doctor may use a tube attached to an aspiration machine (like the suction tool at the dentist) to take out the material.

A D&C is a really quick procedure, but it's also an uncomfortable one, so it will most likely be done while you're under general anaesthetic. Once you're asleep, the doctors will put you in a similar position to the one used for a cervical screening, with your legs in stirrups. By the way, if you're over 25 and you haven't had a cervical screen yet, stick a bookmark on this page and go book your first one, hun! If you've got a cervix, you need to get this test every three to five years.

I've got a red-hot tip for you: if you're booked in for one of the procedures we've covered in this chapter and you also happen to be due for a cervical screening test, ask your doctor if that can be done as part of your surgery. I've done this twice and the doctors have been happy to do it. Saves me the extra trip to

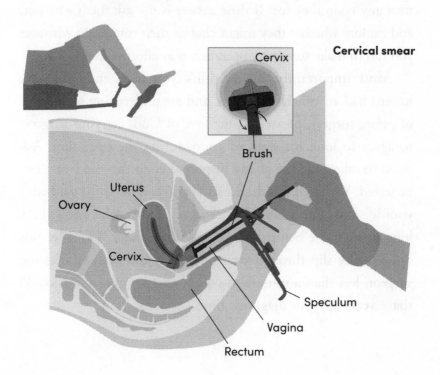

Cervical smear

Cervix

Brush

Uterus

Ovary

Cervix

Speculum

Vagina

Rectum

the doctor, and I'm asleep while it's happening so I don't feel a thing. Highly suggest!

Bottom line: any time a surgeon operates on me, I want them to resolve as many issues as they can in that ONE procedure. If they go in to drain a cyst and happen to spot a load of endo and adhesions while they're there, I want the surgeon to excise those lesions and unstick anything they can while I'm on the table. I don't care if it's not what they thought they'd be doing that day; if I'm under, I want maximum results.

If you've got a surgery scheduled, step one of your prep should be talking to your surgeon about hypothetical scenarios. Ask them what they'll do if they come across any other issues during the operation. If they spot an adhesion, will they remove it? Will they treat any endo they see? If their answer is no, ask them why not, and explore whether they might change their mind. Do whatever you can to make sure every operation is as effective as possible.

Most importantly, if you think you have endo but you haven't had an 'official diagnosis' and are undergoing some form of pelvic surgery, please, for the love of God, get your surgeon to agree to look for signs of endo during the operation. Ask them to take a sample of any suspected endo they find so it can be tested. You need this diagnosis so you can move forward with your life and your health. Once surgery is over, who knows how long it might be before you get another chance. Don't let this opportunity slip through your fingers. It will literally take the surgeon less than a minute to collect that sample, and it could shave years off your diagnosis time.

5

xxx

My surgery
survival guide

You might be a teenager facing your first surgery, or you might be an endo veteran like me, with several surgeries under your belt. Wherever you sit on the surgery scale, I'm going to talk to you as if you're about to have your first surgery because, after reading this chapter, you'll be a whole new type of patient – the sort who walks into a surgical ward feeling prepared, confident and fully aware of what you're entitled to and how things are about to go down. I'm going to share all my secrets, including which drugs I request before going under, how to ask for what you want and how to take control of the situation even when you're shit-scared and wearing nothing but a mesh bonnet and a scratchy hospital gown.

A couple of weeks before a surgery is a good time to start prepping. I like to begin by clearing my schedule for the days after surgery. That way, the only things I have to think about are which movies I'm going to watch and which snack I'm going to eat next.

I suggest getting all the key people in your life involved in your recovery, not just your medical team. Tell your friends and build a network of support around you. If you have a job, book time off and let your boss and colleagues know what's going on. Tell them you will be totally out of action for a number of days and, if you can, give yourself at least two or three more days than you think you'll need, especially if this is your first surgery. This is also a good time to get ahead on projects or contact clients so people aren't hassling you on those days off.

If you're still in school, you'll want to talk to your teachers and organise extensions on projects or assignments a couple of weeks ahead of time. Ask how you can make up any tests or homework that needs to be done. Be clear about the fact you aren't sure how much you'll be able to do while you're recovering. Getting better is a job in itself, and even though you'll spend a lot of time in bed, you're also likely to be on medication and sleeping a lot, so it's unrealistic to think you'll be in the right mental state to cram for a test or write an essay.

It can also be a good idea to let your friends know that you'll be dropping off the radar for a bit to rest and recover. Keep expectations low; you may not be on social media much or feel like answering texts or DMs. If they want to visit you, tell your friends you'll play it by ear after surgery and be in touch if you feel up for visitors. You can't predict how you're going to feel, so the fewer commitments you make, the better. Don't stress about how they'll react; if they're real friends, they'll understand.

Clearing these demands on your time and energy frees you up to feel however you're going to feel after your surgery. It gives you permission to spend your mental energy healing. I get a lot of questions about recovery, and I always say that every surgery has been so different. I might come out of one operation feeling on top of the world by day three, while it takes two weeks to recover from the next one – even if it's exactly the same surgery. Let go of any expectations and try to accept that you'll recover however you're going to recover.

Ask the surgeon

Here are some questions I recommend asking your doctor before surgery. Please go ahead and add any other questions you have to this list. Remember, this isn't you being a pain in the ass. This is part of you being your own advocate. Also, even if your doc seems annoyed by all the questions, who cares! I never let that bother me, and you shouldn't either.

Let's assume you're having keyhole surgery. Here are some questions for you to ask the surgeon:

- How many incisions will you make?
- Where will those incisions be?
- Is there a chance this surgery could end up being an open surgery rather than a keyhole? Why would that happen?
- Will I need a catheter after my surgery? If yes, how long for?
- If you spot any signs of endo or adhesions while operating, will you remove them after you've done X, Y and Z?
- How will the endo lesions be removed?

- Can I request that they be excised rather than burned?
- If you haven't been officially diagnosed with endo, ask this: if you spot anything you suspect is endo, will you take a sample so it can be biopsied? If not, why not? (Press them on this. Do everything you can to get them to agree to take this sample.)
- Can I have my cervical screening test as part of this procedure?
- Can I have something to calm my nerves if I feel scared before surgery?
- Can I have something to calm me prior to waking up?
- Can I have an anti-nauseant before I wake up?
- What might I find difficult to do during my recovery?
- Are there any complications I need to look out for in the days after my surgery?
- Will I be on any medication that makes me dopey or sleepy while recovering? How long will that last?
- How much can I move around during recovery?

Get prepped for the hospital stay

Another way I like to mentally prep is by making sure everything I might want after surgery is ready to go to hospital with me or is within arm's reach once I come home. Being organised helps me feel calm and gives me a sense of control. I've been through these steps so many times that they're practically rituals now, and they put me in a good headspace, so I feel ready for whatever comes my way. Hopefully, they will help you to feel that way, too.

The day before surgery, a pre-admission nurse might call to remind you not to eat anything past midnight or in the morning before your surgery. You can only sip water. No matter how snacky you get, don't be tempted to break these rules and eat. The medication they use to put you to sleep can make you throw up after surgery, and the last thing you want to do is vomit up the sneaky piece of toast and cup of tea you downed that morning. So busted!

Aside from what not to eat or drink, you're not likely to get much more info from the nurse, but that's okay because this is where all of my surgery experience is going to swoop in and save you! As you know, hospitals aren't luxury resorts, so my motto for prepping is BYO everything.

I pack two bags plus my favourite pillow for every surgery. Bringing a pillow might sound a bit OTT, but I promise you'll be glad to have it even if you're only staying for the day. Hospital pillows are as thin as my finger and if you ask for an extra one, you'll be waiting 10 hours and, even then, the nurse will come back empty-handed.

Bag one goodies

- A comfy blanket to go over the hospital sheets.
- Snacks – you don't need to carry a whole esky into the hospital, but a few snacks you love with an ice pack in there will do the trick. I like those little blue freezer bags you can find in most supermarkets. These are some of my go-tos:
  - Jelly cups are the best or you can make a large container of jelly and bring that

- Small cartons of yoghurt or those yoghurt pouches for kids
- Ziplock baggies filled with snacks like energy balls, nuts or freshly chopped fruit
- Small cartons of juice with straws (I like apple juice or Ribena)
- Flat lemonade or ginger ale (good for settling your stomach if the anaesthetic makes you feel sick). I like Coke too, but more for comfort reasons.
- Lollies you can suck on are good because your mouth will be so dry after surgery. I like sugar-free lozenges, Butter Menthols and Soothers . . . they just make my mouth feel better.

Bag two goodies

- Comfy pyjamas with short sleeves – the sleeves have to be short so the nurses can get to your cannula easily without snagging anything
- Woolly socks to keep your feet warm
- Slippers to shuffle back and forth to the toilet
- Bag of toiletries with your toothbrush, face wipes, face cream
- Change of clothes if you'll be there for longer than a day
- Undies – go for granny undies a size larger than you normally wear – you want them to sit higher than your incisions and you don't want them to be tight at all. Honestly, the bigger the undies, the comfier you'll be.
- Laptop and phone
- Chargers

- An extension cord
- Headphones
- Rechargeable heat packs. If heat helps your pain like it does mine, then fully charged heat packs are a MUST. Hospitals aren't allowed to heat up wheat packs or fill hot water bottles for patients any more, at least where I live – it's a safety hazard – so bring at least two rechargeable heat packs so you can rotate them and have one charging while you use the other. If you can't get those, hunt down a few packs of Hot Hands from the chemist. You can lay these right on your chest if you have air pain or wherever it hurts while you're lying flat.

Be warned that coming out of anaesthetic can be overwhelming. You'll feel really dazed and the nurses will be calling your name to wake you up. You may not want to open your eyes, but don't leave them closed for too long or the nurses will start rubbing on your sternum with their knuckles to wake you up. Trust me, you'll open your eyes quickly then because it's so bloody painful. They do this because they need to see your pupils, so just humour them and then go back to sleep.

You might be given an icy pole at this point, but once you get wheeled into your room, ask for your bag, and change into your own pyjamas as soon as you can. Ask someone to stand with you while you change, in case you get dizzy. Even if it hurts badly to stand up for those two minutes while you're changing, do it because you'll feel so much better in your own clothes.

Once you're in bed, chuck a fluffy blanket from your bag on top of the bed. It's a little extra effort but it never fails to make me feel so much better. Around this time, a nurse is going to come in and ask you to eat something. Your throat will be sore from the tube they insert during surgery and your mouth will be dry beyond belief, but they want you to eat something to kickstart the body's systems back into action. They'll offer you a weird little juice and a floppy sandwich, but here's where you can pull out your bag of tricks and eat something you actually like – jelly or yoghurt are good first foods.

From this point, it's time to snack, sleep and watch movies to your heart's content. Be warned that the nurses and doctors will wake you up every two to four hours to take your vitals, check your meds and see how you're progressing. The real rest will happen once you get home. I prefer to recover at home right after surgery rather than stay at hospital, so I'll ask the nurses or doctors to discharge me as soon as I'm feeling well enough to get up and go. I still pack an overnight bag just in case something goes wrong, but my intention is always to leave as soon as possible. Leaving so soon after surgery isn't always recommended and the nurses and doctors don't like it, but I'm more comfortable at home, where I can sleep and take care of myself. For your first few surgeries at least, you should definitely stay a little longer in hospital so they can monitor you and make sure everything is okay. I only leave because surgery has become so routine in my life at this point, it's like brushing my teeth.

Create a calm home environment

When you go for your consultation and book in your surgery, spend some time asking your doctor specific questions. Make sure you take a list with you so you don't forget anything. Ask what your recovery is likely to involve. Is there anything that might be particularly difficult? How might your movement be restricted? Take notes on your phone so you don't forget, and then use that information to troubleshoot your home environment so you can make your recovery as easy as possible.

While I was still living at home with Mum, I came up with this routine that I'd go through before surgery. I've carried it into my life with my partner, Mick, and he's adopted it seamlessly. It might look like a lot, but you don't have to do everything on this list. Pick the things you think might make you feel better, feel free to add your own, and then – about a week before your surgery – start prepping one thing a day that will make your recovery nicer. Trust me, when my room is tidy, smells good and I'm snuggled up in freshly washed sheets, I breathe such a sigh of relief. It gives me room to think, *I can recover now.*

My home recovery routine

Now that I've lived with Mick for a few years, he knows this routine inside out. If I have to work or haven't been able to get everything organised before surgery, he'll tick those last things off the list before I arrive home. I'll walk through the door and my bed will be turned down, electric blanket on, washing done and the house tidy. All I have to do is climb into bed and heal. It makes me feel so cared for.

Pre-surgery prep
- Make the bed up with clean sheets and turn down your side before leaving for the hospital. This way, you can

walk into the house and climb straight into a lovely clean bed when you get home from hospital.

- Download movies to watch and put the remote controls or tablet next to the bed, ready to go.
- Fill any prescriptions for pain meds if you can, and then have those next to the bed with a notepad and pen so you can keep track of when you take them.
- Pop a few bottles of water within easy reach of the bed. Stay hydrated!
- Unwrap about six or seven super-absorbent pads and stick those on some undies, then fold them neatly so you can just grab them and pull them on. The less fussing I have to do with wrappers when I'm feeling sore, the better. I also recommend Libra period pants – they're period undies that are really absorbent and so comfy. They look like nappies but they're actually really good and I was impressed when I tried them last time I was recovering. I'm keen to experiment with other brands and period products as well. They do go up quite high on your stomach, but if you go up a size, they won't put any pressure on your abdomen.
- Hang clean towels and facecloths in the bathroom. I put my towels over the shower door so I don't have to reach or bend down to grab them after a shower. Do anything to make your life easy and stop you from bending over. Even if you think you're overdoing it, you're not.
- Prep your toilet area: put pads, pull-ups and wipes near the toilet so you can easily reach them. If there's a windowsill or ledge next to the toilet, pop a basket on it

and stock it with pads, wipes and toilet paper so you don't have to bend or reach too far.

- Prep some food. It's so easy to go for junk food and takeaways when you aren't able to cook, but it's better for your body if you can eat healthy food, or at least healthy-ish food, while you're recovering. Stock the fridge with some options that you can reheat and prep some snacks. Nothing has to be fancy or take a long time. A day before a surgery, I always cut up a heap of fruit then portion it into ziplock bags that I store in the fridge. Any time I'm hungry, I grab one and take it back to bed. That way I'm resting but still eating well.
- Buy Movicol or another gentle laxative and have it on hand for the first few days after surgery. Pain meds and anaesthetic are a recipe for constipation so you want to do everything you can to keep things moving along nicely.
- Have enough wheat bags on standby so when one cools down, another one is ready to go. If you warm these up in the microwave, remember to always put a mug of water in there with them. If you forget, it smells like popcorn and could potentially set the bag on fire!
- Add anything to this list that makes you feel relaxed, peaceful and comforted: candles, aromatherapy oils, music, a stack of books to read, your dog. You do you, babe.

And there you have it: the recovery routine that hasn't let me down yet. I really hope you don't have to go through this routine as many times as I have but, if you do, at least you'll know that you're doing everything you can to get better. Feeling mentally prepared for recovery is a huge part of the process for me, and I'm positive it helps me bounce back faster.

My go-to bowel prep

Once my physical space is prepped, I prep my body – specifically, my bowels. There's no way I'm risking constipation after abdominal surgery again. Say, for instance, that my surgery is tomorrow but I haven't pooed today or yesterday. I know that I'm going to get an anaesthetic in the morning, then I'll be on painkillers, and since both can stop you up like nobody's business, that means I won't be pooing for at least three days, minimum. My solution is to do a water enema you can buy from the chemist. It isn't glamorous, but it gets the job done. Fleet is the brand that I always use, but I'm sure there are other similar products if you can't find this one. There's so little you can control when it comes to how your surgery is going to go, but this is one thing you can do to make things a little better. Not every doctor will recommend bowel prep prior to surgery, but for me it's the best thing ever. I love knowing I'm going into surgery day with a clean slate.

The first time I encountered a water enema was when I was asked to come in an hour early for an internal ultrasound. This wasn't my first ultrasound rodeo, so I knew what I was getting into as far as that went, but the enema took me by surprise. I arrived early, like they'd asked, and was sitting in the busy waiting room when a nurse came over and handed me a Fleet. It's a clear plastic bottle filled with saline solution, and it looks a lot like that craft glue with the orange lid that kids use.

I wasn't sure what it was, so I asked, 'Do I just sip it?'

The nurse laughed and said quietly, 'No. It's for your bum.' I couldn't believe it when she walked me down the hall to the toilet and told me what I had to do: 'Go in a cubicle, sit on the toilet, then put the nozzle up your bum and squirt all of the solution inside you. Once that's done, get up and walk around and try to hold it in as long as you can. When you can't hold it any more, hop on the toilet and the rest will take care of itself.'

To say this experience was mortifying doesn't even touch the sides. I followed the instructions to the letter and when I could feel that the Fleet had done its job, I sat down on the toilet and all this water came flying out of me. Next thing I knew, I was farting and pooing like never before. I couldn't control any of it, and when someone came in to use one of the other cubicles, I felt bad for them because I couldn't stop it! My soul left my body in horror. After it was over, I walked back to the silent waiting room, positive that everyone had heard everything. I spent the next 15 minutes trying to look normal and avoiding all eye contact. Ever since then, if I need to have an enema before an ultrasound, I handle that at home and I strongly suggest that you ask if you can do the same. If not, at least ask them to point you in the direction of a more private toilet. Good luck!

Day of the surgery

Finally, it's the day of the surgery. You're at the hospital with your bags, sipping water and feeling hungry. Your bedroom at home is all tidy and Zen and waiting for your return. Your bowels are empty. Now, it's just a matter of changing into the hospital gown and waiting to be put to sleep.

That half hour or so while you're gowned up and waiting to go under is nerve-wracking, and it's so normal to feel afraid of what will happen during surgery or worry that you won't wake up (you will!). A nurse will come to put a cannula in your arm for the medications and anaesthetic, and this is when it starts to feel real. Deep breathing and distracting yourself with a podcast or music can help, but if you start feeling really anxious, say so and ask for something to help calm your nerves. I was given Midazolam to calm me down before my first surgery and, if your emotions feel unpredictable and you're spinning into the panic zone like I was, it can help a lot.

Sometimes, the way you wake up from anaesthetic is also unpredictable. Most times, I open my eyes feeling calm and sleepy, but after a few surgeries I've woken up in a full-blown panic – screaming, crying and thrashing around so badly the nurses had to hold me down. They gave me a shot of Midazolam on those occasions, too; I calmed down within minutes and then thought, *Gah! That's embarrassing. I don't know what just happened.* When I asked the doctors if waking up in a panic was normal, I was told that it happens sometimes. So now, before I'm put to sleep, I request to be given something to calm me down *before* I wake up – so I wake up relaxed.

You may not realise that you can ask for medications like this, but you can. The trick when asking for something specific in the operating theatre is to not say, 'Can I have this?' Or 'Is it okay if I have that?' Instead, say, 'Can I please request . . .'

By wording it this way you're making it clear that you, the patient, are asking for something in this procedure. The medical team shouldn't say no to you – not if your request is reasonable. Once you're in the operating theatre, anything you request is documented. If there's proof that you asked for something that wasn't done, someone's going to get in serious shit.

A nurse or doctor might try to brush your request off by saying something like, 'It's okay, love, there's nothing to worry about. You'll be fine.' But their words aren't going to help if you have a panic attack later, so you don't have to accept them. Requesting something clearly and stating your wishes makes it formal. It makes YOU the boss.

Another thing I ask for is an anti-nauseant medication to be administered before I wake up. I can't tell you how many people start vomiting when they come out of anaesthetic. To be honest, I don't know why anti-nauseant isn't administered automatically after these kinds of surgeries. It takes two seconds and it seems like common sense to me. Who wants to wake up from abdominal surgery and start vomiting? Who wants to clean that up? An anti-nauseant is a win-win.

You might feel weird about requesting medications if you aren't a nurse or a doctor but being informed and having a say in how your surgery goes is your right. I make sure things are going to be done the way I've asked for them to be done, and I don't care how silly other people might think my request.

One time, I woke up from a surgery to find that someone had put Vaseline on my brand-new eyelash extensions. (I like to get my lashes done before a surgery because I feel better about myself during recovery when my lashes look good.)

It's standard practice for anaesthetists to tape patients' eyes shut once they're asleep, but by adding Vaseline, they'd clumped up and ruined my new lashes, and I was furious. The next time I went in for a surgery, I told the anaesthetist that I didn't want Vaseline or tape on my eyelashes, and I used very specific language: 'I do not consent to my eyelashes being taped.'

This time, I had a female anaesthetist, and she said, 'That's okay, darling. I work with women every day and I have extensions myself, so I always put the tape on the eyelids.' A dream! Someone who gets me!

But since then, I've only had male anaesthetists. Here's how a recent exchange went down on our way into the operating theatre:

'Excuse me, can you please not put tape or any Vaseline on my eyelashes.'

'I'll try my best.'

'No, no. You will not put them on my eyelash extensions. I had a female anaesthetist who put the tape on the upper part of my lids, and that was fine.'

'Yeah, okay. We'll try.'

At this point, I covered my cannula with my hand and said, 'No, sorry. You're not understanding me, and I'm not going in there until we are both on the same page. I don't want any tape or Vaseline going on my eyelashes.'

Finally, he heard what I was saying: 'Yes, okay. We'll make sure we tape your lids, not your lashes.'

'Thank you.'

I'm not telling this story so you know how seriously I take my eyelashes (very, btw), I'm telling it so you know how to get someone to stop what they're doing and *hear* what you're saying. Surgeons and anaesthetists are busy people with important jobs, and you may not see them much before surgery because their assistants will likely do a lot of the paperwork and prep for them. But, if you want something, don't leave it to their assistant – talk to the person in charge and make sure that they *listen* to what you're saying, that they *understand* what you want and – most importantly – that they *agree* to it. Don't let anyone fob you off with a 'We'll try', or 'You'll be fine.'

Print a copy of my report, please!

Did you know that your medical records from the day of your surgery are yours for the taking? Well, they are, and they're free. You have the right to receive a copy of all records kept during your stay, from your pre-admission forms to the surgical report – a full summary of everything that was given to you, and done to you, during your stay. The hospital can send these things to you after you're discharged.

When you arrive at the hospital and you're at the desk filling in the forms, say: 'I'd like to consent to having all my records printed out and sent to my address.' Guaranteed the person checking you in will be thinking, *Wow, you know you can do that?!*

I think this puts pressure on the people caring for you to do everything by the book even more than they normally would. After the surgery, they'll come to your bedside and say, 'Oh, it all went well, blah, blah, blah,' but they might be inclined to disclose a little more if they know you're walking away with a copy of the surgical report, which details everything that

127

happened while you were asleep. Legally, everything has to be written down: which scalpels they used, which stitches, which medications were administered and when, what they observed inside your body. It must all be recorded, right there in your records.

I found out that these records were available after a surgery to remove an endometrial cyst on my left ovary. When I woke up, I was told it had gone well, but that my right ovary had looked 'a little swollen'. The surgeon didn't seem worried about this; she put that swelling down to ovulation, so Mum and I didn't think much of it either. But I was in so much pain in the days after the surgery that it was clear something was up.

Mum asked an admin person at that hospital for the records from the day of the operation, expecting to have to jump through hoops to get them, but they agreed straight away. They told her that it was freedom of information[28] – all Mum had to do was ask. So, she did. And the notes taken during the surgery included the surgeon's observations: an oversize right ovary, twice the size of the left ovary. Specks of endo, no biopsy done. Everything else looks good. Now, I look at these notes and think, *Hey, doc! Thanks for not bothering with a biopsy! No, really. That's awesome. I'll just hang out and play guessing games for the next few years.*

When another surgeon ended up operating on me to fix the issue, which turned out to be a large cyst in my right ovary, he reviewed the earlier report. According to him, my right ovary

---

28 Department of Health, Australian Government; Office of the Australian Information Commissioner (OAIC).

was 'off-the-charts big', and the dermoid cyst inside it was rock hard. He said, and I quote: 'You couldn't see that and think nothing was up.' That meant the previous surgeon had gone in for one cyst and left another visibly swollen ovary untreated and suspected endo undiagnosed. It was all there in black and white.

Keep good records

Asking for these types of forms is a great step towards creating a clear medical history that you can trace and be clear about what has or hasn't been done, and when. The reality of having endo and/or PCOS is that you are likely to have a long and chequered medical journey. One doctor is not going to cut it, no matter how great they are; I can almost guarantee you'll wind up seeing a number of medical professionals as you search for those who understand what you're going through and can offer new ways of treating you effectively. Over your lifetime, you'll probably see several specialists, surgeons, GPs and maybe physios, acupuncturists, psychologists and natural health practitioners . . . The list will be long.

Whether you're choosing hormone treatments, planning for a surgery or undergoing IVF, one thing that will make this winding road a little easier to navigate is having good signposts. Your medical records are those signposts. Keep them in whichever way suits your life – in a pretty filing cabinet, in multiple folders on a bookshelf, in a cardboard box in your basement, or scanned and saved to the cloud – just keep them! Organising your files chronologically will make them quick and easy to search but do whatever works for you. The key is to keep a paper trail of the treatments you've tried, the tests you've had done, the pills or surgeries that have been effective, and any allergic reactions you've had. When you see a new doctor – which I guarantee you will because shopping around is essential – you'll be able to answer their questions and paint them an accurate picture of your history. This can save you from making wrong turns and wasting valuable time re-trying a treatment that hasn't worked in the past. If you move cities or countries, as many people do these days, good record-keeping becomes even more important.

Good medical insurance is worth its weight in gold!

We can't talk about the admin side of endo and PCOS without digging into insurance because getting shit-hot insurance has been a gamechanger for me. Growing up, Mum only had the most basic health insurance. With three other kids, and me needing surgeries, medicines and specialist appointments all the time, we mostly relied on the public system for my treatments and surgeries. Mum couldn't afford more insurance, and I think that's pretty common. Many people don't have private health cover at all.

But when I got older and had my own money, getting top-of-the-line private health cover became a priority for me. When I was 19, I signed up for really good insurance, and I haven't looked back. I don't want to sound rude or ungrateful because I know we're lucky to have a public healthcare system that any Australian can use, but that doesn't change the fact that I feel I'm better looked after since having private insurance. Unfortunately, that's the way the world works: money often gets better results.

Now, when something goes wrong, I don't have to contend with long wait times for surgeries. I don't have to wait for the cysts growing inside me to get larger or burst before something is done about them. I can be treated by the best specialists in the city and try the treatments they recommend without being ruined financially.

In 2018, I came home after filming *Love Island*. Although I didn't win that competition, I came second (yay me!), which meant I was paid a decent amount of money for the time I was there. The other people I was on the show with were splashing their income from the show on things like cars, amazing holidays and new houses. I had every intention of using my earnings for a deposit on a house, too, but because my insurance hadn't kicked in yet (I had to wait a year before I could start making claims), I ended up paying for several emergency surgeries with my winnings. If it hadn't been for that money, I honestly don't know what I would have done.

If you are in a position to do so, I strongly suggest getting or upgrading to the best insurance coverage you can afford as soon as you can. Make sure that whatever policy you sign up for will cover your endo or PCOS treatments and anything associated with those conditions. If it's likely that you're going to need IVF treatments down the track, make sure the policy includes those as well. These costs can add up like you wouldn't believe!

You'll probably have to pay higher premiums (monthly payments) to get full coverage since insurers don't like agreeing to pay for 'pre-existing conditions', but more often than not, the insurance will pay for itself many times over. Mine has. You never know what's around the corner, and removing financial worry can free up a lot of headspace. I'm no insurance expert, so please ask for help in this area if you need it, and make sure you understand all the fine print before you commit to anything. The goal is to get you the best coverage and the best care, with minimal financial stress so you can get treated, recover and move on to the next thing.

6

x x x

Relationships – the good, the bad and the ugly

One thing I will say in favour of endo, PCOS and the shit-show of surgeries, symptoms and other nonsense that go hand-in-hand with them is that they've helped me to sort the treasure from the trash when it comes to my love life. When everything is going well and you're feeling healthy, it's easy enough to be happy in a relationship. It's only when things are pressure-tested that you find out who people really are.

Unfortunately, nearly all of my partners have come up short in this department. This is worth talking about because – as any person with PCOS or endo will tell you – navigating a relationship (and/or parenthood) while dealing with pain, bleeding, surgeries, hormonal ups and downs, financial pressures and fertility issues is extra freakin' challenging.

Added to this, sex – something that's supposed to be one of life's greatest pleasures – is often painful and unpleasant for endo sufferers and those with PCOS. Put it all together and you've got yourself a recipe for arguments, hurt feelings and nights filled with silence and resentment. I read messages all the time from endo sufferers who are at a breaking point in their relationship. So, it's time to talk about love, lust and the rest of it. As you'll see, my experiences have been as different as night and day.

Night

My very first boyfriend – let's call him Adam (not his real name) – was sweet enough. We got together when I was nearly 15 and he was 17, and a few weeks into dating Adam, I had my very first surgery, so it wasn't like our relationship got off to a flying start. I was laid up in bed with stitches and on pain meds, while he had a driver's licence and more exciting things on his mind. But he turned out to be a lovely guy; he'd visit and bring me snacks, watch movies with me or take me out for a drive so I could get out of the house.

After I made a full recovery, Adam was the first boy I had sex with. Even though my oldest sister had talked to me about her boyfriends, she'd never gone into any detail when it came to that stuff, so I wasn't working with much information that first time. It's not like the sex-ed classes we had at school made things much clearer. I may have learned about anatomy and what the textbook version of things was, but I certainly wasn't walking out of the classroom with a better sense of my body or any idea of what a healthy sex life looked like for me as a young woman. We were all winging it. The first time I slept with Adam, it hurt, which I'd expected from stories I'd heard at school. But the real bummer was that every time after also hurt, and I hadn't expected that. I'd been under the impression that sex was this amazing thing that was so much fun . . . but it wasn't. It always felt sore, scratchy and painful. Definitely not something any sane person would look forward to.

I started wondering if people were lying about how great sex was. It was hard to know since I had nothing to compare it with. When my girlfriends talked about sex, it didn't sound like any of them were having much fun either, so I never bothered to question whether my experience was normal. Like periods, sex was another 'adult' thing that wasn't living up to the hype.

Later that year, I found out I had another cyst and I'd need a laparoscopic operation to remove it. The doctor made it clear that I would not be able to have sex after surgery for between six and nine weeks. On top of the anxiety I felt about what would happen to me at the hospital, I was also worried how the surgery would affect my relationship, how my body would look afterwards, and whether Adam would be willing to put up with another long recovery.

On the night of Adam's 18th birthday, he went clubbing without me. Not only was I underage, I was also recovering from surgery. We'd agreed that I would stay at his house and wait for him to come home, so I was lying in his bed when a text came through from a mutual friend. I could barely stretch across the bed to reach my phone but, when I did, the text said that Adam was making out with someone on the dancefloor of our local club. This was my first experience of heartbreak. I really thought I was in love with him. Even though, rationally, I knew there was never a good reason to cheat on someone, at the back of my mind I couldn't help wondering if that sex ban from the doctor had something to do with Adam's behaviour.

After the embarrassment and hurt of being cheated on so publicly, you'd think I would have stormed out of Adam's house and never spoken to him again. Nope. We stayed together for another year. Only now I was even *more* insecure.

After Adam, it wasn't long before I found myself in another long-term relationship. Let's call this boyfriend Sam. We dated for three years and had lots of adventures together. Once again, I really thought that I loved him – that we loved each other – but sex was still the same old story: sore, scratchy, painful, not fun. Since that was 'normal' in my world, we didn't let that stop us. Sam would get busy for a few sweaty minutes, the way so many guys think they're supposed to (thanks for that, Pornhub), and I'd grit my teeth, pretend to enjoy myself and do my best to hurry things along.

Questionable sex techniques aside, the cysts that kept growing inside me were definitely not making sex any more enjoyable. No one discussed the effects of cysts, or how having one could cause pain during sex. Now I know better. In fact, sex is sometimes a useful tool because I notice that tell-tale pressure right away and can tell when I have a new cyst.

Sam was my boyfriend through two more of my surgeries, and let's just say he didn't win any 'supportive boyfriend' awards after either of them. I had really bad air pain after the first surgery, I was trying not to talk because even breathing deeply was too much, so I was lying flat on my back in bed after taking painkillers. Sam had stopped by for a visit, so he was in the room, too, but he was on his phone. The silence between us was making me feel self-conscious. I wanted his attention, but I didn't know how to ask for attention without being sexual, so I started flirting with him.

Eventually, he asked, 'How long is this recovery going to be?'

'Not long,' I said. As usual, the doctor had told me I was not to have sex for at least nine weeks.

'You know, if this happens a lot, this is why guys go elsewhere.' He said it like this was a lesson I needed to learn.

'So, you think it's okay to cheat?' I asked.

'No,' he said. 'I'm just saying this is probably why men go elsewhere.'

Hmmm.

Should have listened to the doctors

A year later, I was 20 and fresh off my sixth surgery, this time to remove a cyst and treat my endometriosis. It had only been two days since my surgery, but Sam made it clear that he was fed up with waiting. He said, 'If we don't have sex, I'll have to get it from elsewhere.'

That ultimatum hit me at the heart of my insecurities, so, against my better judgement, I had sex with him. I know how insane that sounds, believe me, but for some reason I thought I had to. Just to be clear: me saying yes to sex was my choice. It's true that Sam pressured me. But I agreed to it, so I'm not accusing him of anything here other than behaving like a selfish asshole.

The sex was horrendous (obviously!). By the time he was finished, I was crying and bleeding. He pulled away looking surprised, then said, 'Oh, I didn't realise it was that painful.'

He drove me to the emergency room, and I bawled in the car the whole way, sore and scared that I'd done something terrible to my body, and also SO embarrassed to be going to the hospital with Sam because I knew the doctors would figure out what had happened. Of course, the doctor examining me knew what was up in two seconds flat.

Looking up, the doctor asked, 'Erin, have you had sex?'

'Um, yeah. I have.'

'Why would you do that? You've just had surgery.'

'Oh,' I said. 'I felt like I was okay to do that.'

I can't imagine what that doctor must have thought, or how this situation must have looked. The hospital staff asked if I was okay, and I could tell where they were going with that question, so I made it clear that I hadn't been forced into having sex. While this whole conversation was happening, Sam was standing in the corner of the room. Casual. Scrolling on his phone, not caring – or at least acting like he didn't. I felt so stupid and gross. My legs had swollen up, who knows why, and I was in so much pain.

As awful as this experience was, I rationalised it as Sam not being able to keep his hands off me. I told myself that he'd been too attracted to me to wait for sex. Now that I see things through more mature eyes, it's clear that it was wrong on so many levels: shitty for him to pressure me like that fresh out of surgery, sad that I felt I needed to say yes, and unkind of him to not show me more empathy and care after the fact. If a friend or relative of mine told me a story like this today, I'd be absolutely fuming!!!

If Sam had been a better boyfriend, he could have just laid down and talked to me, brought me a glass of water, watched videos with me, given me a massage . . . Instead, I was tiptoeing around him, trying to keep him happy – scared that my recovery would inconvenience him in some way.

When Sam would sleep over at my house after a surgery, he'd say things like, 'I still have to get up at six in the morning and go to work. You're just going to lie there all day tomorrow.' But it's not like I was ever just 'lying there': I was recovering. A lot of that time, I could hardly breathe without feeling pain, let alone move. I'd lie next to him at night, afraid to turn over in case I woke him up. Instead of asking him to pass me my painkillers in the night, I'd text Mum and she'd creep in quietly and hand them to me. Mum was horrified by the situation and hated the way he treated me, but whenever she brought it up I'd reassure her that things were fine, even though they were far from it. Now, when I think back on all of this, I shake my head and think, *What the actual fuck, Erin?*

Eventually, Sam and I broke up. By that point, I had it in my head that my health issues had been a deal-breaker and I believed that no one would want me because I needed all of these surgeries. Thankfully, that mindset didn't last. As I started opening up to friends, family and people in my online endo groups about the dynamics in my previous relationships, my perspective started to change. Talking things through helped me understand how unhealthy certain behaviours and beliefs were. This brings me to my big takeaway message: If something happens in your relationship that you don't want to tell your friends and family about, that's a sign. That's your gut telling you that the situation is off. Listen to it.

Today, the way I expect to be treated in a relationship is completely different. My attitude has shifted all the way to the other end of the spectrum. I no longer feel that I'm 'too much trouble' because I need surgeries. I never feel that I owe someone an apology for being in pain or that I have to tiptoe around so that I don't disturb them. And I sure as hell don't think you should ever have sex with a person just because they want it. If someone is pressuring you into sex when you know you shouldn't be having it, or if you don't want it, don't fool yourself into thinking it's because you're irresistible. They're selfish and they don't care about you the way they should – plain and simple. It's never worth risking your health or doing something you don't want to do to keep someone else happy. If someone is nudging you in that direction, they're not worth it. This goes for everyone, not just people with endo or PCOS.

From conversations I've had recently, I know that kids are getting into sexual relationships so much younger these days. Believe it or not, there are 12-year-olds out there trying to figure out adult feelings. If it was tough for me to demand respect and set boundaries at 20, imagine how tough it is for them. Nobody was able to help me through these things because I didn't speak about them at the time. I'm speaking now in the hope that someone who is having a tough time in their relationship will read this chapter and understand that things can be different. Whether you are a teenager falling in love for the first time or someone who's been married for 20 years, you have to look at the person you're spending time with and think about how they are treating you. Be honest with yourself. How do they make you FEEL?

Day

Right from the start, Mick was different from other guys I dated. I haven't changed Mick's name because I'll always want him in this book. He single-handedly turned my view of men around by teaching me how it feels to be in a healthy relationship where I'm supported mentally, emotionally *and* physically.

I was 22, fresh off a breakup and going through a man-hating phase when I spotted Mick at the gym. I was instantly attracted to him. In his early forties, he was much older than the guys I normally liked. He was beyond useless when it came to technology and social media (his Facebook profile pic was an emu for God's sake) and completely clueless when it came to dating. He was a few years out of a 18-year relationship with the mother of his three kids.

At this point in my life, things were pretty quiet on the surgery front and my endo and PCOS weren't acting up *too* much. I'd been making the most of this by going out with my mates, having fun and enjoying casual hook-ups. Despite using my go-to flirty tricks on Mick, he was completely oblivious. In the end, I asked a mutual friend from the gym to tell him to add me on Facebook. He didn't. So, I added him. Finally, after a while, he accepted. I waited for him to message me . . . he didn't. I didn't know what was going on; this wasn't the way most guys I knew interacted with girls. Eventually, I sent him a message, which he left on 'read' for more than a week. I was fuming, so I sent another message:

You're going to leave me on read? Go fuck yourself. I'm not going to bother with you.

How do you know I've read it?
Do you not understand how this works?
No.

Mick's cluelessness was actually kind of cute. He thought I was pulling his leg about finding him attractive, and when he realised I actually liked him, he explained that he'd been tied up working on his emu farm and hadn't had phone reception out there. That excuse had my eyes rolling all the way back in my head. *Who the hell has an emu farm?* I thought. *If you're going to lie to me, at least make it believable and tell me it's a cattle farm!* Turned out Mick really did have an emu farm, and he put me off for weeks while he worked out there. I decided to chase him down. I've never chased a guy before, but I was determined to make him see what he was missing out on. We kept things very casual at the start, and when we slept together, it was easily the best sex I'd ever had. I couldn't believe it!

I don't know if it is a generational thing or down to personality, but Mick didn't approach sex the same way I had experienced with guys my age. For one, he didn't see it as a race. To him, sex was something both of us should enjoy. He took his time and knew exactly how to get me in the mood – a first for me. My body responded in a way that totally took me by surprise. Afterwards, I was like, *What the hell is going on here?* It turned out foreplay with a considerate partner I was super-attracted to was the missing ingredient for enjoyable sex. Credit to my nanna by the way, being a fellow endo sufferer herself – she always told me how important foreplay was, and she was so right! Nanna is like my best friend. She may be over 70 but her mindset is the same as mine, and having her in my life made growing up so much better.

Overnight, sex stopped being something I dreaded and became something I looked forward to . . . something I actually *wanted*. Finally, I got what all the fuss was about. I didn't want Mick to get a big head, but I was impressed. So impressed that I was calling up my girlfriends afterwards, like, 'Hey, did you know that this can happen when you have sex?' Most of them didn't, which tells you something.

Since neither Mick nor I were looking for anything serious, we were happy to chat about our experiences and past hook-ups, and we swapped stories with no jealousy or weirdness. But I could tell that some of the things I told him about Sam aggravated and even shocked him. Seeing how he responded to those stories made me think about those experiences differently. It was clear that the things I'd put up with in past relationships were not the type of things all guys thought or did.

We continued seeing each other and having fun until I went away to be a contestant on *Love Island*. By that point, I was starting to like him in a less casual way, but that felt too complicated. It took me going on that TV show and having another bad relationship to see that Mick was an absolute keeper. I was like, *Jesus Christ, this guy is really nice. Too nice!*

When things went off the rails with the new boyfriend I'd met while filming, who did I call to help me? Mick. He was there without question and I suddenly saw things so clearly. About five months after I got back from filming *Love Island*, I snapped him right up and haven't looked back.

Bang on cue, my endo and PCOS really ramped up when we became an official couple, and I had six surgeries during our first year together. Mick took all of this in his stride. Maybe it was because he was older, maybe it was because he'd been in a long-term relationship before me and also had daughters of his own. Whatever the reason, he made it a priority to understand what I was going through as much as he could. He asked a lot of questions, which I really liked, and even came along to a few of my appointments with me.

During one internal ultrasound, he was on the edge of his chair because he could see that I was in so much pain. He kept looking back and forth between me and the technician, then finally asked the guy, 'Are you going to stop?!' Later, he told me that if it weren't for him being with me at appointments like that, he'd never have understood what I go through. These days, he's a full-on endo expert. He's had a crash course and he's passed with flying colours.

One of the things I love most about our relationship is that I never feel ashamed of anything in front of Mick. Nothing is gross to him. If one of his girls has her period, he's off to the supermarket to get pads for her. If I bleed all over the bed in the night, he's whipping the covers off and saying, 'Okay, let's soak the sheets.' One day when I couldn't get out of bed, I taught him how to prep my undies with pads. He stopped when he got to the wings . . .

'Where do these go?'

'Those are the "wings". Wrap them under the sides of the undies.'

'Oh! That's a smart idea!'

A few days after a surgery – the first one I'd had since we'd become a couple – I apologised to Mick for not being able to have sex. I knew he wasn't like other guys, but I couldn't help feeling guilty that sex was off the table. I'll never forget the way he looked at me and said, 'Are you kidding? You've just had surgery, Erin!' I explained that I didn't want him to think we weren't going to have sex for a long time.

'Did you not listen to the doctor, Erin? He said six weeks!'

'And that's okay with you?'

'Yes! Absolutely!'

'Ohhh . . .'

The way he respected those boundaries helped me to frame things in a much healthier way. Recovery stopped being this thing I had to rush through because it was inconveniencing someone else. Instead, me resting and getting better was a priority for *both* of us. I've had many, many surgeries since then, and Mick is still as respectful of this recovery time and thoughtful about how he can support me through it. At night, he puts pillows all around me in bed to make sure he doesn't accidentally knock me in his sleep. If he feels me roll over, he's instantly sitting up, asking what's wrong, checking to see if I need anything.

In the past, my focus had been on how to make sure my recovery had as little impact on my partner as possible. I'd felt so much pressure to 'get back to normal' and find ways of keeping *them* happy even though I was struggling and feeling like my insides were being torn apart. I'd even trained myself to get up and move around right after a surgery so my needs would impact my partner as little as possible.

Mick wasn't having any of that nonsense. I'd go to stand up after a surgery and he'd jump up and say, 'What are you doing?! I'll get it for you.' Eventually, after he had said, 'Erin, STOP getting up!' over and again, it sunk in. Seeing how genuine he was about wanting to help allowed me to accept the fact that it was okay for me to rest and recover. My body needs it. Now, I ask for and accept that help and I don't feel bad about it.

Yes, please pass me the heat pack.

Yes, please bring me my painkillers.

Yes, I'd love you to pick up dinner.

Yes, yes, yes.

Not surprisingly, I recover so much faster now, and I honestly believe this comes down to being in a relationship where I feel free to sink into the couch or bed without guilt. I can rest without drama or pressure. Not having to hide the way I feel or the way I like things to be done is such a relief. As you know, Mick is well trained in my post-surgery routine and he doesn't question it; it's just how we do things.

If Mum picks me up after surgery instead of Mick, I feel relaxed on the way home knowing the bed will be freshly made and ready for me to climb into. He usually calls to find out how we're going, and when I'm 15 minutes away he'll start warming up the heat packs so they're ready to go. Everything will be set up the exact way I would do it because Mick gets that this is my way of having some control over an uncomfortable and unpredictable condition. He knows it brings me comfort, and he supports that 100 per cent.

Sometimes, people who are sick or recovering from a procedure – especially women who are used to taking care of other people – don't like asking for help. They might feel guilty about having their partner bring them cups of tea and snacks and doing the things around the house that they'd normally do. If this sounds like you, try to flip that thinking. Imagine how you'd feel if your partner, parent or child was coming home from the hospital, sore, in pain and exhausted . . . I bet you'd do anything to make them feel more comfortable and you'd be happy to do it. Why shouldn't you get that same care and attention? Let the people in your life help you. It won't be forever, and it *will* help you recover quicker. Isn't that better for everyone?

Partners, please don't give up!

When you're coupled up, whatever's going on with one person affects the other, and endo is no exception. Obviously, the person suffering through endo will bear most of the pressure and stress – not to mention the pain! – but if you care about them, it isn't going to be easy on you either. It's horrible to watch a person you love suffer, especially when you aren't sure how to help them.

Your instinct might be to try to find a way to 'fix' the issue, but endo can't be fixed – it can only be managed. This tension between the sufferer's desire to manage their condition as best they can and their partner's desire to 'fix it' can cause a lot of frustration, miscommunication, resentment and sadness. It's up to each couple to talk about how the woman wants to manage her endo and work out the ways her partner can come to terms with the fact that endo can't be 'fixed' and then support her to manage it.

Your support might look like this:

- Not shaming her for resting.
- Being open to finding more ways of being intimate than penetrative sex.

- Taking on more of the load at home or organising extra help to keep things running smoothly with things like childcare.
- Giving her space to heal or recover in whatever way she chooses.
- Running a bath for her after work.
- Heating up a wheat bag when she's in pain.
- Learning about her condition and going to appointments if she wants you to.

The more you know, the better you'll understand and be able to talk about it.

Endo will put unbelievable pressure on a relationship, but don't let that hold you back if you have it. There are many ways to thrive in a loving, fulfilling relationship with this condition. I know because I'm in a relationship like that now. There are people out there who will understand your situation and take the time to get to know you and your underlying 'stuff'. Remember, everyone has baggage. If you're going to sit there and listen to someone talk about their divorce for an hour, they can damn well listen while you talk about your pain!

If you can't handle it together, handle it alone

Maybe you aren't coupled up, but you want to be. I've spent my fair share of time playing the field, so I know that dating with endo is not the easiest thing in the world. 'I bleed unpredictably' isn't exactly the best ice-breaker. But never forget that there are people out there who will love you and be supportive, so don't accept less. When you think about it, endo is a great way of filtering out the assholes when you're dating because they won't stick around if anything feels like hard work. If you're on a date and doing the whole life story thing, bring up your endo and talk about what it means for you on a day-to-day basis. If they can't sit through 15 minutes of endo discussion, you have all the info you need! Let them go ruin someone else's life.

If things seem to be leading towards sex, but you're sore, tell them straight up: 'You know what, I'm in so much pain today, let's take a rain check.' You might be tempted to add an 'I'm sorry' to the end of that sentence, but you don't need to. I used to constantly apologise for not being able to have sex, but now I stop myself when I feel those words bubbling up. Don't say sorry for something you can't control and didn't choose. It's not your fault.

Chances are, if you're going through a particularly hard time with your endo, you won't have the patience or energy for dating anyway. As nice as it can be to spend time with someone, it can be easier to handle pain on your own terms without having to worry about cancelling on someone or negotiating their feelings.

If you're coupled up and reading this part of the book thinking, *Yeah, right. There's no way my partner would be bringing me snacks or okay with me staying in bed for days on end*, then that's something we should talk about. And this feels like a good time to do that! Regardless of how old you are when you get diagnosed, your endo symptoms are something you're probably going to have to manage at least until menopause . . . maybe longer. Do you really want to face that with a partner who isn't supportive or caring?

I want you to know that if you're in a relationship and not feeling supported, you'll honestly heal quicker on your own than you will having that person around you. Breakups are never fun, but two or three months of feeling shitty and sad is nothing compared with how hard life can be when you're with a person who doesn't understand or empathise with what you're going through.

The thing about endo is that the flare-ups and recovery periods can look a lot like laziness to the outside observer – be that a partner, husband or child. Some days, I'm on the couch with a heat pack down my pants watching telly ALL DAY. Anyone walking by that room is going to think I'm living the life and enjoying a nice day off with my feet up. What they don't know is that I'm burning my skin to distract myself from the searing pain inside. I'd literally rather be doing anything else than lying on that couch . . . but I can't. And because I'm not crying or bleeding visibly, my pain doesn't quite seem 'real'.

This is really tricky in a relationship – especially if you live together or have kids – because your rest might raise eyebrows. When it's time to go food shopping, run a kid to sport or cook dinner, your partner might look at you and think, *How can you possibly be tired? You've been on the couch all day. I've been at work and now I've got to do everything here. Why can't you get up and help?* You can feel that anger and frustration through the house because bad vibes travel through walls. You could even feel so guilty that you might try to get up only to have them say, 'Oh, just go sit back down!' And maybe you'll say thank you and slink back to the couch because that's all you feel you can do, but you know they mean it in a passive-aggressive way, so it doesn't feel good.

Resentment can build up on both sides and create a lot of guilt and tension, so I strongly suggest tackling these issues head on. Tell your partner that you understand how things must look to them, and then try to help them understand why it's necessary that you rest, and how you feel. If it seems like they don't believe you or they're shrugging it off, tell them anyway. Explain how you might be lying there looking still and calm, but inside your body is fighting with itself and you're in so much pain. All you can do is be open about what you're going through and what your body needs. If your partner doesn't understand after that, that's on them, not you.

I read a lot of messages from women who've discovered they have endo later in life. They've been married for 10, 15 or 20 years, and now they need surgeries and rest time to manage their pain. Instead of being able to face those things feeling supported, they're finding out that their partners aren't able to step up in the ways they need them to. So many marriages break up because of the challenges endo brings. Many women put on a lot of weight after years of being on different hormone treatments and surgeries. Some become depressed because they not only feel useless during their recovery, they also feel they look bad to their partner. For some, the lack of physical intimacy on top of the additional pressures on the relationship are too much.

Many of these women feel guilty or angry. Some have left or divorced partners of many years and worry that they aren't going to be okay or that they'll never find someone to love them again. When I read their messages and posts, I applaud them. To me, they're doing better than ever because now they are lighter and freer. They no longer have someone in their home making them feel like they're not good enough.

I honestly hope that you will be able to communicate your way through these challenges and get the love and support you need from your partner. But, if you can't, please remember sometimes it is better to go it alone than be weighed down by someone else. You deserve someone who loves and cares for you as you are, not the way they imagine you could be.

7

xxx

Painful sex – the elephant in the bedroom

Painful sex is so, so common among people who suffer from endo and PCOS – if it's getting you down, it's not just you! And though sex isn't everything in a relationship, it plays a big role in how couples relate to each other. Sixty-six per cent of women with endo FEAR having sex.[29] That's incredibly sad, but I believe it because I see messages and posts on the daily from women with stories to tell:

My partner is making me feel guilty because I'm not able to enjoy sex.

My husband of 10 years is leaving me because I had surgery two months ago and we haven't had sex since then.

Messages like these break my heart. I shake my head and think: *Does that man really think this is fun for her or that she's*

---

29 Endometriosis Foundation of America.

enjoying this? That the lovely, bubbly person he married wants this? He's supposed to love her in sickness and health!

Endo flare-ups, cysts and adhesions can make things painful, but there are also certain sexual dysfunctions that can go hand in hand with endo. These include:

Dyspareunia: Simply put, this just means 'pain during sex'.

Chronic pelvic pain: This one is very vague. It's categorised as 'pain in your pelvis that lasts longer than six months'.

Vaginismus: Causes involuntary vaginal muscle spasms, which can make inserting tampons and penetrative sex painful – in some cases, impossible. Some women have this condition from a young age, while others can develop it later in life due to hormonal changes (i.e. menopause), emotional trauma, or for no clear reason at all.

Vulvodynia: Chronic pain or discomfort around the opening of your vagina. There's no identifiable cause and it lasts at least three months but can also be lifelong.

Lack of vestibular lubrication: Long name for vaginal dryness – especially near the vaginal opening.

Although doctors have joined the dots between these conditions and endo, endo doesn't directly cause these dysfunctions. It's the way that endo takes over the body and causes pain that can *trigger* these dysfunctions. In addition to these dysfunctions that can make sex difficult, it's also important to remember that the pills and medications frequently prescribed for endo also come with side effects – a lowered sex drive can be one of them. That definitely isn't going to help things along in the romance department.

What can I do about painful sex?

Whenever someone messages me to ask for my advice in this department, I always explain that dealing with painful sex is a long game – one that has to be played *together*, as a couple. Sadly, it's not as simple as sex being painful when you have a cyst or adhesions, and sex being awesome once those have been treated. That can happen, and if it does – great! Go get some and enjoy it! But if sex doesn't get better after treatment, then see your gynaecologist and try to get to the bottom of what might be causing the pain.

Ask your doctor about the conditions I just described to see if those symptoms match up with what you are experiencing. If sex still hurts after any underlying physical issues are addressed, then it's time to look at something called the feedback loop. Whenever your body experiences pain, your brain logs that memory and draws a link between whatever activity you were doing at the time and that pain. So even if there's no physical reason for pain during sex any more, your brain is still on high alert. The next time your partner makes a move, instead of getting turned on, your brain can jump to emergency mode and activate a protective response in your body. Muscles that would normally relax in anticipation of something pleasurable will lock up shouting, 'No, no, no!'

That means you won't feel aroused, your body won't produce any lubrication and your vaginal muscles will tighten to the point that sex is painful, only for totally different reasons this time. Your partner might find it hard to understand how something that was easy and fun before is suddenly difficult. They might say, 'Oh, okay. Well, let's just go slow,' but slow sex can still be painful, it's just SLOWER!

Even if sex is great after you recover from endo surgery, there's a risk that adhesions will eventually develop and rain on that parade. At one point, my right ovary was stuck to my bowel, which was stuck to my bladder. It was a mess in there! I wasn't bleeding, but sex was so, so painful – worse than anything I'd experienced before. When the doctors figured out what was wrong, they explained to me that during sex, things sort of move around naturally inside the female body. Adhesions prevent that natural movement. But if you try to show your partner where it hurts during sex, and you are pointing to your hip or way off to one side of your abdomen, they might be confused because that's nowhere near your vagina. It can be hard for them to understand what the hell is going on.

All I know is that too many women with endo and PCOS are saying yes to sex when they don't want it. They're thinking, *Fine. Let's get this over and done with.* But what's the result? More pain! A stronger feedback loop! A lot of us have done it to keep a relationship alive, but this mindset needs to change because it's not right and if it keeps happening, there's a good chance your sex drive might say, 'Fuck this' and go AWOL altogether. When that happens, you'll stop having sexual thoughts, feelings and desires. The idea of doing laundry will be more appealing to you than sex, and *this* is when relationship problems can really kick off.

In the past, when my sexual desire has packed up, I've noticed that it's around the same time I'll start fighting with a partner. It's not because I'm angry that we're not having sex but because I'm *aware* that we aren't having it. If they try to crack a joke about the lack of sex, instead of laughing and agreeing with them, I'm more likely to be overly sensitive about it and react in a not-so-great way that creates more tension.

Sadly, these types of problems don't have easy fixes. Some partners might be understanding for a while but get bored of being patient and start demanding sex. Other partners might understand, but they might also withdraw all other forms of attention and intimacy until your bond is broken beyond repair. This type of tension and pressure can wear people down and cause the type of conflict that eventually leads to a breakup. But it doesn't have to be that way.

Talk it out

Communication is the key when it comes to navigating any issue in a relationship, especially the issue of painful sex. Talking about sex isn't something a lot of us are great at doing, but it's important because it can help avoid resentment and lead to other options – there are so many other ways to pleasure each other besides penetrative sex. It doesn't have to be all or nothing. And if your partner isn't willing to talk through the options and figure out a way to work around this issue, maybe they're not for you.

My hope is that younger generations will be more patient and understanding with each other when it comes to this because they will have grown up with access to more information than older generations. They'll have a better understanding of endo and the potential issues. On top of that, talking about sexuality and feelings is becoming more and more normal – it feels like things are moving in the right direction.

One thing you can try is to bring your partner to a few of your appointments. Sometimes, having a doctor in a white coat explain the science behind what you're experiencing makes it more concrete and real for them.

Figure out what feels good for YOU

This approach – specifically foreplay – worked wonders for me, so I'm going to encourage you to give it a red hot go. Retraining your body to enjoy sex and working out how you can enjoy it is something that can absolutely be done, but again, it requires having a partner who is up for trying new things and patient enough to understand that it might take time. The more you can tune in to your body and be more selfish when it comes to your sex life, the better. I don't recommend being selfish all the time, of course, but when it comes to sex, you've got to be in it for yourself as well. The more you like sex, the better it will be for you AND your partner. After all, people who don't enjoy sex don't want to have it!

Whatever your age, there's nothing to be ashamed of when it comes to getting to know your body and figuring out what makes YOU feel good. Lock the bedroom door and muck around with yourself – you'll find out what works for you. Everyone has their own sex language, so spend some time working out what yours is and experiment a little. Ideally, learn as much about sex and about your own body *before* you get intimate with a partner so you don't end up suffering through years of painful sex like I did.

There's nothing wrong with googling things you are curious about if you feel too shy to ask someone, but look on sites or platforms that prioritise female pleasure because that's where you'll learn about techniques that work for women. Porn sites aimed at men are full of moves that don't feel so great to be on the receiving end of for many people. Too many boys and men get all of their information about female pleasure from porn. That's why, when they hook up with a woman in real life, they go crazy trying to do all this weird stuff at once, and it's like, EWWW! Stop! Slow down! The lady in the movie might have looked like she was enjoying it, but that's called ACTING! She's getting paid.

Once you know what turns you on, you'll be able to show or tell the person you're having sex with. If they're a halfway-decent person they'll be grateful! I reckon the majority of people want to walk away from sex thinking their partner enjoyed the experience, so if someone isn't rocking your boat, help make them better!

It took me years to discover what an orgasm was. I figured, *If he's done, I must be done.* I had no idea! Because sex was so shit, I'd often get drunk beforehand because I figured I may as well be numb for it. I'd be all 'Woo-hoo!' at the time because you don't feel as much pain when you're drunk, but wow, I'd SUFFER the next day. Thankfully, I found a partner who knows what foreplay is, takes his time with it and knows how to turn me on and give me an orgasm. Lo and behold, I discovered I could be completely sober *and* have the best sex of my life.

Even though I've learned to enjoy sex, it's still painful sometimes, but the big difference is that I don't suffer in silence anymore. If something hurts, I speak up and we hit pause to either try something different or come back to it another time when I'm feeling better. Sometimes, I might be sore but I'll also want to have sex – so we will. And I might feel fine and have an orgasm, but then afterwards I'll be in heaps of pain. Other times, I might have zero pain, but then I'll get turned on and suddenly feel really sore because now my ovary is aching . . . my poor body doesn't know what's going on!

The bottom line is that you deserve to have a healthy and enjoyable sex life; it just might take a while to work out how to achieve that. A flexible approach is the key – have sex and enjoy it when you feel good, and hold off when you aren't up to it. If you're in a relationship and the moment isn't right, that might mean saying, 'I don't want to be touched right now, but I'll touch you.' Or it might mean explaining that you aren't up to being sexual that day. Intimacy can be expressed in other ways. It will be frustrating for both of you at the start, and from time to time, but if you're communicating openly, then anger and resentment are less likely to sneak up on you.

Common treatments for sexual dysfunctions

Depending on your diagnosis, your gynaecologist may prescribe counselling or cognitive behavioural therapy (CBT) to address that feedback loop we talked about earlier, or other psychological and emotional issues that might be factoring in to make sex painful. Often, people will put up with painful sex for years before seeking help, so there can be a lot of baggage to unpack.

A doctor might prescribe vaginal dilators for a condition like vaginismus or dyspareunia. These are basically penis-shaped tubes that come in different sizes from small to large, and the idea is you use one a couple of times every day to gently 'stretch' your vagina gradually until you can tolerate a larger size without pain. Good times, huh!

Another thing that might help is enlisting the help of a sex therapist or attending couples therapy together. These aren't roads I've been down myself, but I absolutely would try them if I needed to. If you love someone, and want to make things work, learning how to communicate effectively is well worth a shot, and it's a skill that could improve all areas of your relationship, not just in the bedroom.

Therapy and dilator treatments take time, patience and consistency, and they have varying degrees of success. I haven't tried these therapies, so I can't speak about them from experience. All I can do is let you know that these are some options on the table, and possibly worth exploring with your doctor.

Botox (yes, really!)

Some solutions to painful sex are a little less conventional. A while back, I got a message from a woman who shared something that had worked for her. She had vaginismus, which made having sex way too painful. Thanks to a suggestion from another woman in the same situation, she decided to try Botox – not in her face, but in her vagina! It worked like a charm for her, and now, once a year, her gyno puts her under and injects Botox into the vaginal muscles that spasm. Within a week, those muscles are fully paralysed and unable to spasm, which means penetration (for her at least) is pain free. She credits this treatment with saving her marriage and helping her to enjoy sex again. How good is that!

Botox isn't going to be a magic cure for everyone but, for certain women, it is an option to explore. Like any procedure, you've got to talk through the pros and cons with your gynaecologist to work out if this treatment is a good choice for you. The procedure is usually carried out under local or general anaesthetic as an outpatient procedure. Doctors who offer it say it usually takes about four to five days to recover, with the Botox coming into full effect one week after the procedure. In some cases, the injection alone will be enough to allow for painless penetration. In other cases, this treatment might be combined with the use of dilators and therapy. I haven't had it so I can't say what it's like personally. I'm simply sharing because I've heard good things – and I want you to have options so you can be your best sexy self.

8

xxx

Life can still be
an adventure

There are days where you just can't. Can't drag yourself out of bed. Can't run that errand you said you would. Can't pick up the phone to send that birthday text. But despite all the struggles and challenges endo throws your way, life can still be a series of adventures – amazing ones – if you can use those times when you *are* feeling good to go and chase them down.

You never know how adventures are going to unfold. When I finished high school, my goal was to become a nurse. I assumed that would be my only career, but I also ended up appearing on reality TV shows and then growing a social media presence. I never saw either of those two things as ways of earning an income, but sometimes life drops opportunities in front of you that are so far from what you have in mind for yourself. It's up to you to grab those opportunities with both hands and see where they take you.

When I was 18, I randomly saw a casting call on Facebook for an Australian version of an American dating/makeover reality

TV show. I applied on a whim. It sounded crazy, but I thought *Why not? I'm not doing anything that can't wait.* When I rocked up to the dodgy industrial building the producers had rented for the auditions, it crossed my mind that it might be a kidnapping ring rather than a legit television gig. Thankfully not. To my surprise, I was comfortable in front of the camera, and I ended up being cast for the fifth season of *Beauty and the Geek*.

I'd had a few surgeries by this point, and I was super self-conscious about my body – especially the long scar from my first surgery – but this felt like an exciting opportunity, and they were going to fly us to Fiji to film the show, so I was definitely in. Just because I was cast, though, didn't mean that my insecurities suddenly vanished. The other girls on the show had these great bodies and they didn't have to worry about things like bleeding unexpectedly or dealing with pelvic pain. They also didn't have scoliosis like I did – a condition where the spine curves differently from the norm. It starts in puberty and there's no cure, you just have to manage it (sound familiar?). I thought that I looked a bit funny in clothes because one shoulder sits higher than the other, even when I'm sitting up straight. Just another thing I worried about! I wasted a lot of my energy during filming worrying that my scoliosis would be noticeable on TV, or that I didn't look as good as the other girls. As much as I liked the experience of being on the show, I wasn't able to enjoy it as much as I could have. You know the annoying thing? I've seen pics of me sunbathing with my 'geek', Nathan (such a lovely guy), and I looked fine! I wish I could travel back in time, grab myself and say, 'Don't waste your time worrying about your body. Enjoy the ocean! Enjoy Fiji! Enjoy these people!'

I came back from filming that show with a tan, some prize money and some new friends. I had no expectations that going on the show would lead to anything afterwards, so it was straight on to the next thing: becoming a nurse.

Love Island

A few years later, fresh from a breakup and in the thick of my 'man-hating' phase (except for Mick, I liked him!), a friend sent me a link to a casting call for the first series of *Love Island Australia*. She said I reminded her of a girl on the UK version of the show, and that I should go for it. I'd just had my boobs done, I was feeling good, and I had nothing to lose by trying – so I sent an application in. I didn't give it a second thought until the production team got in touch a few weeks later to ask me to submit a video and then audition in person. Two auditions later, I was on the show. I think they liked that I was relaxed in front of the camera and not afraid to speak my mind.

I was really enjoying studying as a nurse, but the prospect of lying in the sun for seven weeks with a bunch of people my age *and* getting paid for it was too good to pass up. I quit my job and flew to Spain, ready for some fun. Most days my pain wasn't bad at all. The pace of life was so relaxed, and all I had to do was hang around the villa and chill with people. All the girls were in bikinis for most of the show, and because sudden and unpredictable bleeding was a constant worry for me, I had to figure out how to manage it.

To avoid turning the villa's pool into a bloody crime scene, I started wearing tampons 24/7. If you're wondering whether that's a good idea, it's not. Doctors have told me flat out that tampons are not only very drying but also that wearing them constantly – especially when you're not on your period – can destroy the good bacteria in the vagina. I hadn't heard of menstrual cups back then, and it's not like I could have gotten away with wearing a huge pad in my sexy swimsuit, especially when I was surrounded by cameras at all times. What's a girl to do?

BEATING THE BLEEDING BLUES

I have to confess that I still go through phases where I wear tampons every day to prevent accidents even though I know I shouldn't. I haven't tried using a menstrual cup yet, but I will. So many people rave about them, and apparently once you get the hang of using them you never look back. I worry about how they would cope with my flow, but I promise when I get around to trying one, I'll put the full report on my social media.

I've also become a big fan of those Libra period pants I mentioned in Chapter 5. They look so good with high-waisted pants, but another reason I love them is because I can wear them instead of a tampon just in case the blood starts flowing. With these, I pull them on the second I get out of the shower every single day and there's no drama. I feel so secure, and I love knowing that I'm going to be okay – that I'm not going to leak, and these pants aren't going to bunch or slip the way a pad can. But, as much as I love them, I think we can all agree they wouldn't have done me much good poolside on *Love Island*!

Coming off *Love Island* was a very different experience from my first TV show. *Beauty and the Geek* aired seven months after we were finished filming, so I was able to watch the whole show with the rest of Australia as it aired. That was my first lesson in the power of editing, and how producers can twist words and build a non-existent narrative by cutting unrelated footage together.

The episodes of *Love Island*, on the other hand, would be aired 24 hours after filming. To me, that was part of the appeal when I signed up: they wouldn't have time to edit that dramatically – or so I thought. But the downside was that the show would air while we were in the villa, so we wouldn't know how it was being received until it was all over. Even so, it felt like an okay gamble. It was a new show; how many people would even watch it?

Suddenly social

The second I landed in Spain the producers of *Love Island* took my phone away. At that point in my life, Instagram was just another app I liked using sometimes. I didn't have a social media strategy, I didn't follow any influencers, or anyone with a blue tick, and I didn't spend any time thinking about what content to post. Since it was the first season of the show, none of the cast had expectations of growing their following or becoming social media personalities. We'd all signed up to do the show for the same reasons: to travel to Spain, live in a mansion for seven weeks and maybe find romance.

Once we were in the villa and filming, we weren't thinking about our social media accounts. When someone new came into the group, we'd be all over them to find out what the latest song was, or which celebrities were dating. 'How many followers do I have?' was the last thing any of us would have asked.

These days, people are so much more media savvy. They've seen what can grow from appearing on a show like *Love Island*, so when they sign on as a cast member, they have a game plan and they're there to build their personal brand.

Seven weeks after entering the villa, I was given my phone back to find that my Insta following had exploded from a thousand or so followers to over 300,000 while I'd been on the show. *Love Island* airs in so many countries around the world, and I couldn't believe that so many people were that interested in the show, or in following me. It was shocking, honestly.

I remember the producers pulling us aside and telling us not to read the comments on our Instagram posts – they were worried we'd be upset by the floods of negative comments we'd been getting after certain storylines had aired – but how could we not read our comments? I scrolled back through my timeline and quickly found out that my persona on the show was 'that girl who argues all the time'. This really bothered me because

I knew that a lot of my fiery reactions to people on the show had been more about me still being upset and angry at my long-term boyfriend over our breakup rather than whatever some castmate had done or said. I just wasn't dealing with my feelings the right way. But once I had a little more time to process that perception of me, I made peace with it by reminding myself that most people argue, they just don't have cameras filming them around the clock.

Since it was impossible to defend myself against comments that were weeks and weeks old, I just thanked my new followers for watching the show and moved on. As surprising as it was to find myself with so many followers, that in itself has turned out to be such an adventure, too – one that I'm enjoying and finding a lot of meaning in today.

The power of social media

At first, I found being a 'public person' on social media terrifying. Every time *Love Island* aired in a new country, I'd get a load more followers (and heat!). When people came at me in the comments, I'd fire back. A lot of people respected the way I stuck up for myself, but others didn't like it. I'd get messages from parents telling me I needed to act like a role model. But why? I didn't nominate myself as a role model, and if their twelve-year-old was watching *Love Island*, then that's on the parents, not me.

Once I realised I didn't have to change who I was, I was able to make my social media my own space. When I signed on to appear on the sixth series of *I'm a Celebrity . . . Get me out of*

Here! I chose Endometriosis Australia as my charity. I figured even if I didn't win, I'd at least have a chance to talk about endometriosis, and people watching who didn't know what it was might google it and learn something.

We filmed the show in the South African jungle, which was pretty awesome. But the best thing about the experience was being able to talk openly about my endo and PCOS in such a public way for the first time. I'd had one ovary removed five weeks before leaving for the jungle, so I was feeling really good about my health at that point. I was optimistic about my future and enjoying the idea of finally being able to live with no more bleeding. That's what I thought, anyway.

When I explained what living with endo was like to a few people in the camp, I was blown away by how interested and sympathetic my fellow cast members were. They were shocked by some of what I shared – most of them weren't aware of how many people suffer from endo, or how it impacts them. Later, when I was out of the jungle and watching replays of the show, I was so touched to see that Miguel Maestre (who ended up winning) got emotional in the hut when talking about my endo. He has daughters, plus he's just an amazing, sensitive man, and hearing what I was going through really affected him. It meant a lot that he, and the rest of the cast, took the time to listen and take it in.

When I had an endo flare-up halfway through my time in the jungle, because I'd explained it to the others, I didn't have to hide the fact that I wasn't feeling great. I was bleeding a bit, so I went back to my tampon routine. The jungle is bad enough on its own – you're already peeing and pooing into a long drop with spiders and snakes – so having to fuss around with blood and tampons added a whole other layer I really could have done without. I was afraid to spread my legs for too long in case something from the jungle flew up there!

After completing the scariest challenge of all time with Ryan Gallagher and Myf Warhurst where we'd had to slide off a huge cliff in a dingy (honestly, go watch the clip of that challenge on YouTube), I had a classic endo clot moment. As we were walking back to camp, I was feeling really proud of myself for getting through the challenge when I felt a familiar flash of pain in my abdomen. I looked down and, lo and behold, there was a big old blood clot right there on the ground. I stared at it while Ryan, Myf and a lovely crew member called Darren, who had also been part of the crew on *Love Island*, stopped walking. They were shocked because there was a lot of blood, and immediately started asking if I was okay. It all seemed so out of place in that jungle setting that I think I was a little shocked, too.

I mumbled something like, 'Yeah, that's nothing!', then my brain switched straight into clean-up mode. I picked that clot up and chucked it into the jungle for the wild animals, then took off one of my boots and used my sock to wipe down my leg as best as I could.

I knew we still had to get through a bit more filming that day, so I turned around and shoved the sock in my underwear – pretty much up my vagina – adjusted my shorts, then told the three of them that I was good to go. My khaki shorts weren't in a good way, but I knew the director would shoot to avoid showing viewers the stains. People at home might be happy to watch us eat impala anus and bull's testicles for a bush-tucker trial, but they'd riot if they were shown blood from a vagina. I had no doubt about that.

Myf, Ryan and Darren were so good about the situation; they didn't make the moment any more awkward than it already was. We got back to camp, announced the results of our challenge, and then I walked straight to the hut to let the production crew know that they were going to need to bend the show's rules and wash my clothes for me. It was going to take a lot more than a bucket of cold water to get those shorts camera-ready.

From that day on, I was in a lot of pain. And with very few painkillers and no wheat packs or Hot Hands, it wasn't the most fun. The on-set medical team offered me Panadol, but I told them I wouldn't bother unless it was something stronger.

Everyone in the camp contributed in lots of little ways to help me feel better, and I appreciated that so much. Miguel in particular was so sweet. He'd boil water for me and fill up my metal drinking bottle so I could use that as a makeshift hot water bottle, and he kept the pot on the fire so I could top up my bottle whenever it cooled. People worried that my skin was getting burned by holding the bottle on my skin, but I explained that it was fine because I didn't feel the burning inside that way. To them, that sounded extreme but, as you know from the chapter on pain, to me it was so normal.

Eventually, the producers gave me a proper hot water bottle with an animal print cover since we were in the jungle. I kept it stuffed down my shorts all the time. When Mick watched from home, he spotted it peeking out of my shorts a few times and realised I must be having a flare-up. I didn't get much time on camera in the last few days because as interesting as endo might be to talk about, it doesn't make for great TV. I was just walking around with a hot water bottle and sleeping a lot. When the time came to leave the show, I was so ready to get back to Mick, my dogs, my bed and my wheat packs.

Community is a beautiful thing

Being on *I'm a Celebrity* . . . brought a lot of new people to my social media accounts, and I noticed right away that most of these new followers were from the endo community. I loved that so much because for many years, online endo groups had been a lifeline for me. Knowing that I could open my laptop and talk to women all over the world who understood exactly what I was going through was always so comforting. When I was younger and my friends would be out partying while I was at home waiting for a surgery, I'd go online and nine times out of 10 there'd be some woman in Denmark or India or America who was having the same surgery the next day. Instantly, I'd feel less alone.

I still rely on these groups when I have a question about a treatment or I'm weighing up the pros and cons of a certain surgery. If you don't belong to an online group, this is the part in the book where I push you gently but firmly towards joining at least one. I promise you there's an amazing sisterhood full of information, support and understanding waiting for you. Even if you join and never post anything, that's okay! Reading other people's posts and comments will help you so much – I guarantee you'll benefit in some way. Personally, I like Facebook groups because you don't get comment trolls in the same way as on open platforms like Insta. I've popped the names of a few of my fave groups in the Notes section at the back of this book to get you started. (Do it! Do it! Do it!)

Once I had more of an endo community behind me, I felt empowered to pull the curtain back on the other side of my life. Until then, I'd kept my posts limited to the fun side of life; my pages were full of pics from parties, my dogs and cute outfits because that's what I thought everyone wanted to see. Then one day, I was lying on the couch covered in heat packs, feeling sad and in a lot of pain, and I thought, *Let's post this and show people how it really is.* I got a great response, especially from people who knew exactly how I was feeling, and that meant more than putting up a sexy pic you know is going to get likes (I still do that too, though!).

People love seeing something that's real and raw. They appreciate the honesty, especially on a platform like Instagram where most accounts only show highlights. I want my page to reflect all sides of my life – good and bad. If I try a new hormone pill, and have a terrible experience, I'm going to post about it. If I find a new product that I think will make life a little more comfortable for my endo and PCOS sisters, I'll share that, too.

I get a lot of shit for sharing my experiences because people feel strongly about certain treatments. For example, I posted about my experience of taking Zoladex, which is a hormone treatment used for people with breast cancer or prostate cancer. It tells the brain to stop producing luteinising hormone, which triggers ovaries to produce estrogen. Essentially, taking six-monthly injections of Zoladex put my body into a temporary early menopause. Dr Manley's hope when suggesting this treatment was that it would stop my cysts from growing – possibly in the long term – and hopefully help my endo symptoms as well. In the short term, it worked. My ovarian cysts did slow right down, but it hasn't solved anything in the longer term.

The comments were heated because Zoladex and a similar drug called Lupron are both under the microscope in the US for having terrible long-term side effects. Some people didn't like me highlighting this drug as a treatment option, but I wasn't promoting that drug or even recommending it. I was simply telling people that I was trying it out and sharing my experience of how it felt to me.

Turns out, being on that treatment was torture! By month two I was calling up Dr Manley to tell him that I hated him because my hot flushes and mood swings were out of control. Eventually, I finished the sixth and final treatment and posted about that too. I think the more information we share with each other, the more we'll have to work with when it's our turn to make tough decisions about our health. Being open about what we've gone through is better for all of us.

I get DMs and messages constantly from women looking for advice from someone who's been there, done that. I love helping in any way I can. But I also want to make sure I keep a balance so my Instagram is a place where people can see my life as it really is: relationships, drunken nights out, endo pain, family, dogs, barbecues, surgeries. My endo is a part of me, just like your endo is a part of you, but it isn't *all* of me and it isn't all of you. We're so much more.

Let's be kinder to ourselves, okay?

Being on a TV show has a way of making you very aware of your appearance, especially if you aren't feeling your best going into filming. And it's not like most of us need an excuse. Weight and appearance are front of mind for many women; that's just a fact.

My weight has gone up and down since I was that chubby kid with high cholesterol, and when you're short, like I am (5 foot 1 without heels), even a little extra weight can look like a lot. Not only is weight gain a classic symptom of PCOS, it's also a common side effect of most hormonal treatments. It's hard to escape that double whammy. After going on my first diet planned by a nutritionist in my early teens, I developed an eating disorder where I basically didn't eat much at all. I lost a lot of weight and thought I looked great, even though my friends and family would later tell me they thought I looked sick.

Throughout my late teens and early twenties, my weight went up and down depending on whether I was recovering from surgery, trialling a new hormone treatment or in a relatively healthy place. But in my mid-twenties, as the number of treatments and surgeries I was having increased, my relationship with my weight got worse. In 2019, I had five surgeries and, even though I struggled to stay healthy at the beginning of that year, eventually I surrendered to the trackies. I started drinking more, ate shitty food and stopped doing most physical activity. I felt so sore, and so unhappy with my weight, that it was exhausting. I gave up. That summer, I thought, *Fuck it! I don't care anymore.*

But the thing was, I DID CARE. I cared a lot! So much so that I let my feelings about my body stop me from enjoying life.

On the days I wasn't in pain, I still didn't go out. I didn't go to the beach with friends, I didn't sit out in the sunshine and there was zero chance you'd find me in a swimsuit. If I went in the pool, I'd wear Mick's shorts and T-shirt. I hid away because I was so down on how I looked.

I turned down invitations to go out at the last minute because I had nothing to wear. I'd start getting ready for a night out, but most of the time I'd wind up crying in the cupboard because nothing fit me properly. If Mick came in to comfort me, he'd try his best to help by suggesting I go shopping and buy clothes in another size. I'd say, 'THERE IS NO OTHER SIZE! You don't understand!' I had it in my head that I had to be a certain size. Anything else was unacceptable.

I was unhealthy inside and outside, but mostly in my head. I was trapped in a vicious cycle where I'd feel sore so I wouldn't exercise, then I'd feel bad about that so I'd eat shitty food, and then I'd gain weight and feel even worse. The craziest thing is that when I look back at pictures of those times, I looked fine! That seems to be how it goes for me – maybe you, too. It's easier for me to see myself more clearly and be kinder in hindsight than in the present.

When the offer to be a contestant on *I'm a Celebrity . . .* came through, I was just starting to come out of this phase. I said yes knowing I was the heaviest I'd ever been, but I decided that since I didn't know the people I was going into the jungle with personally, it didn't matter what they thought of me. I put it out of my head that people would be watching me on TV and judging my body. Also, raising awareness and money for Endometriosis Australia seemed like a great way to wrap up the crappy year on a more positive note.

A few days before leaving for the jungle, I took a 'before' photo knowing I'd lose weight while I was away because the food would be so bad. Once I got out of the jungle, I took an 'after' photo and, as predicted, I was considerably lighter. I put both pics on Instagram with a caption saying I couldn't believe I'd let myself get to my 'before' photo size.

People started sharing their thoughts about my 'before' body right away: *Wow, Erin you put on so much weight.* Because I'd already lost that weight, I could take those comments, and I could handle watching myself on TV when the episodes aired. If I had still been carrying that extra weight, it would have been so hard for me to deal with.

But what blew me away was that there were way more comments scolding me for the way I perceived my 'before' body:

Don't talk about your body like that!

Your body just went through all of those surgeries, and now you're criticising it!

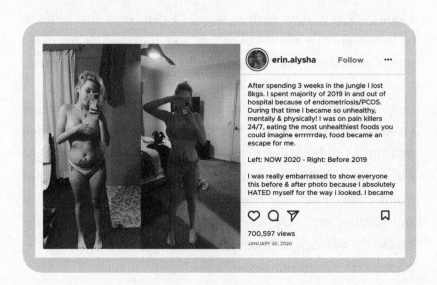

erin.alysha   Follow   •••

After spending 3 weeks in the jungle I lost 8kgs. I spent majority of 2019 in and out of hospital because of endometriosis/PCOS. During that time I became so unhealthy, mentally & physically! I was on pain killers 24/7, eating the most unhealthiest foods you could imagine errrrrrday, food became an escape for me.

Left: NOW 2020 - Right: Before 2019

I was really embarrassed to show everyone this before & after photo because I absolutely HATED myself for the way i looked. I became

700,597 views
JANUARY 30, 2020

I scrolled through those comments and it dawned on me that these people were so right! I was always looking at my body through a lens of 'fat' or 'not fat'. Maybe it was time to see it through a kinder lens.

As much as I understand why people keep dieting and exercising despite their pain, I do think there's a point where we can push ourselves too hard. I've been that gym bunny smashing it on the cardio machines, but it's a hard routine to sustain long term, especially when dealing with unpredictable health issues. When you're lying on the couch barely able to sit up, the last thing you can think about is working out. It's hard enough to do when you're feeling 100 per cent healthy!

The challenge is endo and PCOS pain, and the medications that treat those conditions, have a way of tipping the hormonal balance against you. The most common side effect of most hormone pills is weight gain. And PCOS often goes hand in hand with thyroid problems, which adds even more hormonal and metabolic issues to the mix. If chasing the perfect body is your goal, you're fighting an uphill battle. Even if you do achieve the body you want by pushing yourself to the physical limit or dieting your way to 'skinny', ultimately, you might still lose. All this dieting and exercise can cause flare-ups potentially leading to another surgery and a new pill that could throw your metabolism into turmoil again. The older you get, the harder this battle gets to win.

I'm only 26, but already I'm finding that weight won't come off as easily as it used to. When I started exercising again and saw no results, I thought, *Hang on! What's going on here?* At 19, I could eat whatever the hell I wanted while recovering from surgery then go back to my gym routine and have abs again in no time. Not now. My body has been through too many hormonal ups and downs. Gone are the days of eating a cheeseburger from Maccas first thing in the morning. Back then, I'd order one salad a year and think I was so healthy!

These days, if I gain some weight while I'm recovering, my body hangs on to it for a long time – up to a full year. I've had no choice but to adapt to this new reality by taking the focus off working out (it feels too hard most of the time) and putting more focus on eating mindfully. Not only has this been working for me, but it also feels like a much nicer way to treat my body when it's going through so many shitty things.

It's all about balance, babe!

There is a lot of online chatter about how to manage PCOS and endo through diet, and while there are probably benefits to some of those diets, I haven't had success with any I've tried. But hey, if following a regime to the T is your thing, I'm not here to say don't do that. Same goes if you love working out or doing sport; if that brings you happiness and makes you feel good – keep going! Maybe you can even skip this part of the book and come back to it another time. But if you're struggling with the body issues I just spoke about and you're finding it hard to feel motivated to eat well or exercise, this is the section for you!

You can relax, because I'm not about to tell you that you need to eat perfectly all the time or work out X number of days a week. Far from it. I've murdered my soul drinking apple cider vinegar every morning, and I don't want that life for you! I hate reading books that tell me to stick to a certain diet; I honestly believe that you're better off getting savvy about healthy food swaps and controlling your portion sizes.

It's taken me a while to find what works for me when it comes to maintaining a healthy weight and feeling good, but it's my food choices rather than exercise that gets me there. So, here's my big suggestion . . . wait for it . . . put your focus on eating healthy-*ish*.

That's it! No fad diet, I just want you to aim for healthy-*ish*. That might mean eggs on toast in the morning instead of fast food. A chicken wrap for lunch instead of chicken and chips, flavoured water instead of soft drinks. Nothing crazy.

It was a 10-week health challenge during a COVID-19 lockdown that kickstarted this change for me. One friend of mine who happens to be a personal trainer was running an online course, and another friend was doing it. She wasn't a gym junkie at all, but she was meal prepping, losing weight and toning up. Since I had time on my hands, I signed up. Imagine my shock when the meal plan turned out to be awesome! Mick and I were eating pasta and burgers – just with a few ingredient swaps. Those alternatives tasted more or less the same as the ingredients I'd normally use, so my mindset around healthy eating completely changed. The numbers on the scales started shifting, I felt much better in myself and it finally dawned on me: I can still eat food I like *and* be healthy. It doesn't have to be all or nothing.

The app to keep you on track

I am about to sing the praises of an app called MyFitnessPal (MFP). You've probably heard of it; you may even have it on your phone right now. If not, I suggest you download it ASAP. It's free, it's easy to use and it's honestly the most useful healthy eating tool I've ever had. (I'm not getting paid to say this, by the way.) I reckon the best feature of the app is the barcode scanner: hold your phone camera up to the barcode on any food packaging and all of the nutritional info is instantly logged on the app.

I started using MFP when I was on my lockdown fitness kick. At the time, I was tracking everything because I was keeping eye on my total calorie intake, but I quickly got curious about other aspects of my nutrition, like how much sugar, fat, fibre or salt I was eating. I know a lot of people don't like tracking their food, and I understand why – it can feel like an extra job – but tracking, even for a week, really can start to change how you think and feel about the food you're eating.

And here's the thing I want you to know: you don't even need to track consistently or stick to a certain calorie count to benefit from using this app. I don't use the app daily anymore, but every now and then I'll track a few days of eating, just to see how things are looking. I find this helps keep me mindful, not only when it comes to how many calories I'm eating, but also in terms of the quality of my food.

One of my food obsessions is an HSP (halal snack pack), which you can buy from kebab shops. It's a box of deliciousness: mixed kebab meat, chips, garlic sauce, barbecue sauce with five extra cheeses . . . It's so amazing that my mouth is watering from describing it. The first time I entered an HSP into the app I nearly screamed. It came in around 3000 calories and was loaded with sodium, fat and sugar. Talk about a reality check!

That didn't stop me from eating and enjoying it, but it did make me determined to eat much lighter, healthier food the next day. You don't have to say goodbye to comfort foods; you just have to be realistic and work around them.

I was also shocked by the amount of sugar and salt that are in a lot of the things I thought were healthy. When I worked out that my go-to yoghurts were full of sugar and calories, I swapped to Greek yoghurt with a drizzle of sugar-free maple syrup (tastes so good!). It didn't feel like a big sacrifice at all, but those small daily changes added up.

Next on the hit list were my soft drinks. Me and soft drinks were a thing – we were in a long-term relationship, but as I scanned those barcodes day after day, I couldn't deny the numbers. My sugar intake was off the charts and the calories from these drinks alone were crazy. Gradually, I started weaning myself off them. I switched to sugar-free soft drinks at first, then I switched to flavoured fizzy water. Not going to lie, giving up soft drinks was really hard. I know that makes it sound like I was coming off drugs, but I was addicted. Lemonade was my drug of choice; I drank it with everything. Now, water and coffee are the only things I drink during the day. This one swap alone has been huge. I'm less bloated and I know I've dropped weight because of it. After a surgery, I will treat myself to a sneaky lemonade or Coke and it's always so good! But after that I'm back on water.

I also find tracking useful when I'm feeling a bit shit and I don't know why. Flicking back through a few days of food entries shows me when I've had too much of a certain thing or too little of something else. I'll think, *I haven't eaten much fibre in the past couple of days, that's probably why I can't poo.* It helps you spot those patterns and adjust accordingly.

I love using this app in the supermarket because if I see something that looks good, I can scan the barcode, and say 'Nup!' if the nutrition turns out to be garbage. If you're craving a certain snack, the app will help you choose the best version of that snack. I might look like a weirdo standing in the aisle scanning barcodes, but I don't care. I want to eat popcorn while I watch *Titanic*, not a salad!

So, there you go. That's my hot take on health! Forget fad diets and killing yourself at the gym. Rely on healthy-ish food choices and MFP to get you to a place you can feel good about *and* sustain over the long term. If you don't know much about nutrition or would like more guidance about healthy eating, book a consultation with a nutritionist or consult a personal trainer. There are always people who can help.

Most of all, be kind to yourself and take a longer view of life. If this year is going to be a tough one health-wise, focus on getting through it and feeling as good as you can so you can recover. Next year can be your year of fitness. It doesn't have to happen now. And if you've been on the couch for seven days eating junk because you're in pain, it's okay to put that week behind you. Beating yourself up about it won't help or change anything. Your best strategy is to go into next week with a goal of eating better. Life is too short to be unhappy in your body year after year, and it's too long to deny yourself the foods you love. Find the middle ground and stick there.

9

xxx

The world has babies on the brain

Content warning: I'm about to talk about fertility issues but my comments may not be what you expect. I do not want to have a baby, so this chapter explores fertility issues from that point of view. I know that this is not how many women feel, so if you are in a tough place with fertility or struggling to conceive, you might want to skip this section. I don't have advice for people trying to conceive, though I have watched women in my family go through these struggles. My suggestion is to lean on those endo groups I told you about earlier. They are literally full of women going through similar things; you can learn so much from their experiences and find great advice that will help you. Please know that I'm sending you love on your journey and I hope that your dream comes true. ♥

Picture this: you're a teenager fresh out of your first surgery for an ovarian cyst. You're lying in a hospital bed, out of your mind from the pain and your surgeon walks in. He spends two minutes talking about your recovery before launching into something that sounds like this: 'We're going to start you on this hormone pill because we want to preserve your fertility and make sure those ovaries are working. If that doesn't go well, we'll spend the next few years trying these 700 medications. Some of them have pretty bad side effects and might make your kidneys burst, but hey, at least you'll be able to have a baby when you grow up!' Okay, that's not exactly what they'll say, but you get the idea.

Meanwhile, you're sipping on a juice the nurses gave you, thinking, *Wait a sec, I don't care about babies right now. Can we talk about my body? The pain I'm feeling, will that stop soon? Will these stitches in my abdomen leave a scar? Am I going to need another surgery? Will I grow another cyst? When can I start playing soccer again? Will I be better in time to go on that trip with my mates?*

You're young. You're focused on the NOW. You want to know if your life is going to be pain free and enjoyable next week, next month, next year. The doctor is looking 10 years into the future. The doctor has babies on the brain – *your* babies. Why? Because you're (almost) a woman, and women have children. That's the way of the world.

Looking back, I wish my fertility hadn't been a topic of conversation in that recovery room. I was 14 for God's sake – still a child myself. I'd like to say this was a one-off, but it wasn't. Pretty much every time I've had surgery on my ovaries throughout my teens and early twenties, the follow-up conversations included a warning that I might struggle to get pregnant or a heads-up that I'd likely need IVF one day.

Never mind that motherhood was the very last thing on my mind after having these surgeries – I just wanted to feel better and hang out with my friends.

It's true that endo and PCOS can make it harder for a woman to conceive naturally, but this is often one of the first things we're told when we're diagnosed. Of course, it's something that needs to be discussed, but as a teen and a young twenty-something, it would have been great if my doctors had spent more time talking to me about my treatment and recovery rather than my fertility. At 17, I was told that I'd need to try for a baby between the ages of 23 and 25 if I wanted kids. I wanted to be living life with my friends, not looking for a guy to knock me up because I was on a baby deadline.

I've always felt that the expectation that I would have a baby (or at least *want* to have one) has played too much of a role in the care I've received. So often I've been frustrated by doctors who've chosen to protect my fertility over helping me resolve my pain – even when I've made it clear that I'm more concerned with fixing my medical problems than I am with having a child.

A few years ago, a female surgeon in the public system who'd operated on my ovaries a couple of times refused to operate on me again because one of my ovaries was so damaged. There were cysts growing on that ovary constantly and it was very thin. When it became obvious that it needed to be removed, she cut me loose because she didn't want to be the one to do it. She felt strongly that it should be preserved for the sake of my fertility.

I assured her that having a baby wasn't something I wanted. I was really suffering from the pain that this ovary was causing, and I begged her to treat me. Not only did she refuse to operate, but she also told me she couldn't think of another doctor in the city to refer me to. I felt furious and let down by her. Eventually, I found another surgeon to remove the damaged ovary, but my situation didn't improve much because I still had one troublesome ovary left.

Going against the grain

My remaining ovary had issues – a lot of them. It grew cysts at a shockingly fast rate, and all my doctors seemed to agree that pregnancy was not going to be an option for me – definitely not naturally. I wasn't a good candidate for IVF either because the hormones I'd need to stimulate egg production would also send my cysts into overdrive. I'd be in hospital with a burst cyst long before a viable egg could be retrieved.

I am totally okay with not having a baby. As much as I think kids are amazing, and I love all the children in my life, I don't feel maternal in the slightest. Family doesn't have to be biological, and life can still be full and amazing without being a parent. Mick was already a father to three great kids, so there was no pressure from him. All I want is to find a solution that will improve my symptoms and pain in the long term. Life is about making choices and then living with the consequences. Yes, my biology has influenced my decision not to try to get pregnant, but it's still *my* choice and I don't feel sad about it. Far from it. I know it's the right choice for me.

I don't feel like less of a woman because I'm not going to have a child, no matter what the rest of the world thinks about it! From every direction, I get bombarded with the message that I have to have a baby in my arms before I will be accepted as a 'real woman' or allowed to make decisions that limit my fertility.

If Mick and I are at a barbecue or party and babies happen to come up, at some point, I'll say, 'I can't have kids' or 'I'm not going to have kids' and things get so awkward. Even after I say that it's my decision not to pursue motherhood, people still either pity me or refuse to accept that I know my own mind. They'll say things like 'Never give up' or 'You can adopt' or 'You're too young to make this decision. You'll regret it when you're older.' Look, adoption is awesome, and if I wanted to be a mum I'd be all for it. But that's not where I'm at. Maybe I will regret not having kids one day and I'll deal with that when the time comes. Let *me* worry about that.

I am aware that the way I feel about motherhood is not the way many women feel, but thankfully there are doctors who are willing to go to great lengths to help women with fertility issues have a baby. Having watched a relative go through it, I know that it can be a very long and painful journey, not to mention an expensive one, but it can work. If you're reading this and you want kids, GO FOR IT! I fully support you in your choice, just like I hope you support me in mine.

When it comes to women's healthcare, there should be room for all of our feelings and all of our choices. We go to gynaecologists for the health of our reproductive organs, but there's so much more to reproductive health than just fertility. In my case, being healthy means not spending another year of my life recovering from surgeries that don't make me better. It means not gritting my teeth through another internal ultrasound. It means not cancelling plans because I can't get out of bed. I've already lost my teens and most of my twenties to these diseases, I'm not willing to give up any more decades. Quality of life NOW is more important to me than being a mother, and I believe I should be just as supported in my choice to pursue the surgery to remove my second ovary as a woman who wants a baby is to pursue IVF treatment.

If you want to preserve your fertility at all costs, work with your doctor to do that. Make sure they are choosing treatments for you that support that goal *and* help you feel better. If having kids is not something you want, then make sure your doctor knows where your priorities lie. Push them to see you as more than a 'potential mother' and encourage them to try treatments that will deliver an outcome that YOU want, not the outcome that society wants.

I spent a couple of years struggling to find a doctor who was a good fit for me. The end goal of my doctors always seemed to be for me to have a child; my end goal was to live pain free. I needed someone who was going to be on my team.

Drastic times call for drastic measures

Many surgeries and a couple of burst cysts after my first ovary was removed, I walked into Dr Tom Manley's office for the first time. One of the walls in his office is covered with photos of babies he's delivered. The babies are adorable, and Dr Manley has seen a lot of their parents through hormone injections, egg retrievals, embryo implantations, as well as some miscarriages . . .

I imagine seeing that wall of tiny faces gives his new patients hope that they'll get their baby one day, too.

As nice as that wall might be to look at, adding a face to it is not *my* dream. Far from it. What I want, more than anything, is freedom from my reproductive organs. I'm sick of being held hostage by them. That's honestly how it feels. I've spent the last 12 years doing everything my doctors have asked of me. I've gone under anaesthetic for surgery over and over again. I've been for every scan they've requested and I've tried every hormonal treatment put in front of me – no matter how extreme. Not one of those things has made my life better in the long term. It's my turn to call the shots now.

I believe that having my remaining ovary removed will improve the quality of my life. When (not *if*) that ovary is removed, my periods will stop forever. No ovary = no more cysts. No more random bleeding. No more nights spent on my hands and knees while a cyst bursts inside me. No more putting my body through the ordeal of anaesthesia and recovery only to have a new cyst pop up days or weeks later.

There's also a good chance that this surgery will improve my endo symptoms. I'm aware that there's no 'cure' for endo – I know there's no guarantee – but there's a strong possibility that it will slow the growth of my endo. There's a chance that I will have less pain – maybe a lot less. Instead of having multiple surgeries a year, I may only need surgery once every few years to remove the endo or unstick adhesions. That's good enough for me.

This is why I've been asking . . . NO . . . *begging* Dr Manley to 'deliver' my ovary for years now. I never let him forget that this is my endgame. If he rings me up and happens to mention that he's just delivered a baby, I say, 'Cool. Can you deliver my ovary, please?' He laughs, but I'm dead serious. I've even told him he can stick a photo of it on his wall. It won't be as cute as those newborns, but it will be a dream come true for me.

As much as I hate the way that my fertility is often prioritised over my quality of life, I understand that doctors like Dr Manley spend a huge chunk of their careers treating women who are desperate to be mothers. Every day they sit across from couples who would give anything to have a baby, so when someone like me comes to them wanting to shut down that possibility, they're reluctant to act.

Unlike all the other doctors I'd seen, Dr Manley didn't rule out removal of my second ovary as an option. I knew he wasn't keen on the idea, but he said he'd consider it once we'd tried other treatments. This was further than I'd ever got with any other doctor, so I was willing to work with him. Dr Manley was the first surgeon who seemed to hear me when I told him that living a good life now was more important to me than my ability to have a child in 10 years' time.

When Tom wanted to try me on Zoladex, which triggers medical menopause, to see if it would slow the growth of my cysts over the long term, I was fully against it because I knew the side effects could be pretty severe, and the prospect scared me. But in the end, I gave it a go. It did slow my cysts and improve things for a while, but within five days of coming off the medication, it was clear that more cysts were growing, and we were back to square one.

Frustrated, I called Dr Manley to talk about my ovary (again!): 'Fuck's sake, Tom. When you're in there next time, can you please just take it all out and chuck it away?' He laughed and said it wasn't that simple. Then he told me to come in for an appointment.

The top of the roller coaster

I decided that I was ready to go in to battle for what I wanted and do whatever was necessary to make this surgery happen. I brought Mum to the appointment with me, and when Dr Manley saw us both, he joked that I'd brought back-up. I replied, 'It's not for me, Tom. It's for you.'

I told him I knew that he'd done everything he could to avoid getting to this stage, but that we had arrived. I was crystal clear that I wanted my ovary removed – and soon. I said I'd even be willing to go through the egg retrieval process so he could feel happy that I had some eggs as back up for the future. But, once he had those, I wanted everything else out. I told him I hoped he could do it because I trusted him and didn't want to go to someone else, and that my mind was made up. To my shock, he said yes.

I sat back, stunned. 'Wow! I had a full argument planned in my head, and now you've just said yes straight away so I don't know what to do!' Dr Manley agreed that he'd tried every avenue to avoid removing my ovary, but that it was my best option now. Together, we laid out a three-stage game plan that would take place over the coming weeks. As a compromise, it would include a few steps to preserve my fertility (for his peace of mind, not mine).

1. We'd start with another keyhole surgery to unstick my adhesions and remove any new endo. Dr Manley would also take out my left fallopian tube, since it was floating around in there without an ovary attached to it. I'd start taking hormones to stimulate my ovaries and grow as many follicles as possible. The more follicles I could grow, the more mature eggs they'd (hopefully) be able to harvest. Those hormones would likely trigger new cysts, so they'd have to keep a close eye on them to make sure they didn't grow too big. I told him that was fine, but I refused to have another internal ultrasound. The last one had been so painful that I just could not have one more.

2. Two weeks after the first keyhole surgery, Dr Manley would go in again. This time, he'd remove all the cysts that would have grown because of the stimulating hormone, then he'd harvest as many eggs as possible. There was no telling how many there would be. I might have 19 follicles but only one viable egg. I told him he would have to see it as a 'lucky dip' and be happy with however many eggs he got. I didn't care whether he froze them, fried them or scrambled them. They were purely to tick that 'fertility options' box for him.

3. A couple of weeks after that second stage, Dr Manley would perform another surgery to remove my remaining ovary and fallopian tube. He'd leave my uterus and cervix intact to give me the option of carrying a baby if I ever wanted to try that route in the future. He said it was

possible that I might be able to carry a baby but that my small pelvis and scoliosis would likely make it a very painful pregnancy. He wasn't selling me on the whole pregnancy thing. But again, leaving these organs ticked another box for him in the 'fertility options' checklist, so I was happy to agree. The most important thing was that my ovary was finally coming out!

With my ovary and fallopian tubes gone, there wouldn't be anything in my body to produce estrogen, so I'd probably go into 'surgical menopause' (menopause induced by surgery). When Dr Manley brought this up with me, I reminded him that he'd already put me through menopause once, and I was prepared to do it again.

I knew that I'd need hormone replacement therapy (HRT) to replace the missing estrogen from the ovary, and that there were risks to being on that medication in the long term – risks that would likely show up in my late forties or fifties. But again, I was okay with that. I'd been on so many pills already, and besides, have you ever read the side effects of a birth control pill? There's no such thing as a 'risk-free' treatment when it comes to hormones.

I assured Dr Manley that I was all-in. I explained that I'd rather be happy during my twenties, thirties and forties and deal with health challenges later in life than live the next 30 years the way I'm living now. I already feel like an old lady and I'm only 26. I'm bed-ridden many of days, and there are a lot of things I can't do because of pain. If I have this surgery but end up having health challenges later in life, oh well! At least I'll be able to say I lived life to the fullest and did all this cool stuff when I was young. Bungee jumping, travel . . . whatever!

We booked the dates for my procedures, and I was so, so happy. Floating-on-air type of happy. When I got up to leave, Dr Manley mentioned that I looked as though I'd lost weight. He was right, and I told him it was because I'd been in so much pain lately that I hadn't been eating very much. I'd been coming home from work, taking pain meds, then going straight to bed so I didn't have to be in pain.

He said, 'Well, that's no good.'

'Exactly, Tom.'

Hope feels good

In the days after that appointment, whenever I was in pain, I'd think, *I've got to remember this because pretty soon I won't feel this type of pain. Life is going to be so awesome.* But first, I had to tick another box. This time, it was an appointment with a professor of gynaecology – one of the best in the city. Turns out it isn't enough to give your surgeon permission to perform this surgery, you also need to prove that you are capable of making this decision and a prime candidate for it.

Having to prove you are worthy of having surgery that could potentially relieve the chronic pain you've been living with FOR OVER A DECADE is some real bullshit if you ask me. I guarantee the only reason it's required is because I'm a woman who doesn't want her reproductive organs. It's as though my decision is so 'out there' and so 'unacceptable' that I must be crazy!

Honestly, my decision feels like the most logical one I could make in this situation. It's not like I'm a teenager with one surgery under my belt saying, 'Take it all out! No kids for me!' I'm an adult who has already lost one of her ovaries. I have a less than 10 per cent chance of having a baby, even with IVF. I've endured so much. This is not a decision I'm making lightly.

The consultation with the professor cost me $310, which is a lot but I paid it because it felt like a small price for my freedom. As much as I wanted to walk into that woman's office, throw myself on her couch and say, 'Get this fucking ovary out of me, I'm so over it,' I knew I couldn't muck around. I couldn't give her an opportunity to say I was too angry or not in the right mental state to make a balanced and informed decision about my own fertility. The stakes were too high. I *needed* her to be on my side.

It makes me so angry that we have to go through things like this. If I suddenly announced that I was pregnant next week, do you think anyone would insist I attend appointments with professors to certify that I was stable enough to be a good parent? No fucking way! People would be sending me balloons and teddy bears and asking exactly zero questions.

As frustrating as all of this was, I kept it to myself. My new life was so close I could practically see it. I was even willing – no, excited – to go through the egg retrieval process because I felt I'd be able to help other women going through it in the future. I knew I wouldn't be able to relate on an emotional level because going through an egg retrieval when you're desperate for a child is way more intense, but at least I'd be able to talk them through some of the practicalities and help them understand what to expect.

For the first time, I was sitting at the highest point of the endo roller coaster – at the top of the biggest loop. From there, the view was amazing. I could see the next 30 or 40 years of my life and they were mostly pain-free and beautiful. I could picture being in my thirties and actually enjoying my life! Travelling, working, having adventures with people I loved without the constant presence of endo and PCOS. I couldn't wait to see how my body responded to detoxing from pain meds. I even felt excited to walk past the period care section in the supermarket and think, *No more bleeding for me!*

I found myself wondering what I'd do with my time and energy once pain wasn't sucking so much from me. What new things would I be interested in once my brain wasn't dominated by all this endo-anxiety? What would it feel like to leave the house without worrying that I'd bleed or have a blood clot? What would I fill the space in my head with? I couldn't even imagine. The world felt bigger. There was so much . . . potential.

Back down the roller coaster

The thing about getting to the very top of a roller coaster is that it's a long drop down. One step into our three-step plan, I noticed a few missed calls from Dr Manley while I was at work. When I rang him back, I could tell from his voice that it wasn't going to be a good call.

He started by saying that he'd had several sleepless nights over the past week, and that he'd gone back and forth with other medical professionals, discussing my situation, but the end result was that he wasn't going to go ahead with the egg retrieval process after all.

I was okay with having one egg retrieval process, but I wanted it to be a 'lucky dip', where Tom would go in and get as many eggs as he could, and he'd have to be happy with whatever he got. But the professor I'd seen wanted me to have two retrievals – she didn't feel one would be enough. But now Dr Manley didn't think that putting my body through the hormones needed to prepare for a retrieval was the right thing to do; he didn't think it was safe. And without that egg retrieval, the ovary removal was off the table. As you can probably guess, I didn't take this news very well.

Dr Manley went on to explain that there was another issue in play: the other doctors involved in my case felt that my ovary was functioning well enough as an estrogen factory for my body to warrant keeping it. They felt that if I were to go on hormone replacement, the risks of me having a heart attack when I got older were too great. Dr Manley said that he'd pleaded my case, but it wasn't enough. He was so apologetic, but I didn't care. I didn't want apologies – I wanted surgery. He'd given me his word that he would take my ovary if I went through the other steps. I'd held up my end of the bargain . . .

I've watched *Botched*, so I know that there are surgeons out there who will give you horns on your bloody head if you sign on the dotted line. They'll cut your tongue in half so you can look like a fucking lizard fairy if you pay them. But when it comes to my body? Nope! Sorry. We're going to make you keep that ovary that's causing you so much pain.

For what? So I can have a natural source of estrogen and live longer while suffering? I was in disbelief, and was only half-listening when Dr Manley suggested that we try a new treatment, a hormone pill called Norimin-1, for four weeks to see how I did on that. 'What if I grow another cyst while I'm on that?' I asked. 'Will I need another surgery?'

'Yes. Probably.'

Don't even get me started on the fact that every surgery I have is a risk. Keeping my ovary will likely mean that I need to have many more surgeries. I could die on the operating table in any one of those surgeries, yet somehow that is a risk these doctors are willing to take over me (maybe) having a heart attack when I'm 50. When do I get a say in my own life?

I was back at the start, riding the roller coaster.

10

x x x

What now?

If the last chapter proves anything, it's that I still don't have this figured out. Just like any other endo warrior, I'm out here doing the best I can. For a few weeks, I honestly thought I'd nailed this thing. After years of shit experiences, a great surgeon had finally agreed to give me a treatment I believed would improve my life. I was buzzing! I shared my good news with my family, friends and work colleagues. I posted about it on social media and soaked up all the lovely messages from people who were so happy for me – *I* was so happy for me! The anticipation of living a more 'normal' life had me glowing. It didn't matter if this wasn't a cure because a reduction in pain and surgeries was going to be a huge improvement in my books.

But, as you know, the plan changed. And now, like so many other people with endo and PCOS, I'm trialling a new hormone pill for a few weeks and managing my symptoms and side effects while working a busy job and also trying to be a good partner, friend and daughter.

As frustrating as this set-back has been, I'm certain I'm going to have the ovary removal surgery – and soon. I'm going to keep looking until I find a surgeon to help me realise my goal. I thought I'd found that in Dr Manley, but no. Don't get me wrong, I still think he's an excellent doctor, and I know that he's helped hundreds if not thousands of women, but he wasn't able to deliver the results I need, so it's on to the next one. I'm not waiting around for him to change his mind. I have a life to live.

I am hopeful that when I do have my reproductive organs removed, I'll have similar results to my nan. When I read posts from women who've had these surgeries and they say they haven't needed to have endo removed for about 20 years it gives me hope. It may not work out like that for me, but if it could, that would be so awesome! In 20 years' time, maybe I'll write another book about how it feels to live free from pain. I hope I get that ending. I hope we all get that.

Even though we still don't fully understand endo, where it comes from, how best to treat it or how to cure it, I love that it's becoming more visible and more talked about. People are so much more open about their experiences of living with it, and by raising awareness about how hard endo is to live with, they're doing all of us a favour. Awareness benefits everyone in the endo community because the more people understand what we're going through, the more they'll care about the issues relating to it and the more supportive they'll be.

Never be afraid to add your voice to the mix. It's okay to talk to your boss or colleagues about endo – help them understand your situation so they can support you when you need it.

Let people help you if you're having a bad day or recovering from surgery. Ask for more work flexibility if it will reduce your symptoms. When people with endo can feel more supported in every aspect of their lives – work, love, play, parenthood – then we really are getting somewhere.

Science will catch up, eventually (I hope!). Endo research is still miles behind other diseases, and endo only gets a fraction of the funding that other diseases get. Even though a similar number of women suffer from endo and diabetes, endo gets just 5 per cent of the money that diabetes gets.[30] That's a pretty insane funding gap, and you have to wonder why. Obviously, diabetes is serious and can be life-threatening, so that explains some of it, but could the fact that it's a disease men also suffer from explain the rest of this gap? Hmm, I don't know. You tell me!

In the UK, there's five times as much research done on erectile dysfunction, which affects 19 per cent of men, than PMS, which affects 90 per cent of women.[31] There seems to be a theme, that's all I'm saying.

Whatever the reason, endo's profile is growing and funding for scientific research into endo seems to be going up alongside it. The Aussie government allocated $15 million to funding endo in 2018 and 2019,[32] and in 2020 they spent another $9.5 million on five research projects dedicated to improving diagnosis and treatment, and understanding why we get endo in the first place.[33] It seems like the more we talk about endo, the

---

30 *Pain and Prejudice.*
31 *The Guardian.*
32 Ibid.
33 Department of Health, Australian Government.

more money it gets, so let's keep this going by speaking up, sharing our experiences and adding our voices when we can.

I'm going to keep sharing my experiences – bad and good, publicly and privately – so that women coming after me have as much information as possible. If you want to know what the latest research is saying, or if there are any new treatments being trialled, trust me, women in online endo groups are going to be talking about those things way before your GP even hears about them.

That's why I'm all about the endo sisterhood. We have each other's backs, not to mention a unique bond. Just the other day a woman came in to get a vaccine when I was on shift and I saw that she had endo listed in her medical history. I got so excited when I saw that. I pointed to her paperwork and said, 'Same! I have endo, too. We're twinning. How are you going with that?'

'Not too bad right now. How about you?'

'Ugh, I'm dying today. So much pain!'

'It does suck, doesn't it?'

It was just a little moment in the day, but it felt good to connect to a stranger like that. Endo *does* suck. It sucks on several levels, and that woman knew exactly how much.

I hope that this book has given you a similar feeling and made you feel less alone as you deal with whatever it is you're going through. I also hope that I've given you an idea of what might come your way so you can go into situations more prepared than I was. Sometimes, being mentally prepared is half the battle.

Most of all, I hope this book gives you the confidence to be strong and speak up for your wants and needs in *every* area of your life, not just the doctor's office. If you haven't already joined an online endo group, this is the last time I'm going to remind you to do that. I promise you'll never regret it. You'll learn so much from the amazing people there, and more importantly, you'll never, ever be alone in this situation. There will always be someone online who can relate to whatever you're going through. Come say hi if you see me blowing up a comments section. You know I'm always up for an endo rant.

Thank you

Firstly, I would love to say a huge thank you to my close friends – you know who you are, my favourite four. An ever bigger thank you to my mum, Anabela, for coming to every single surgery I've had. You've been the best. I love you! To my partner, Michael, my biggest thanks for being extremely supportive and understanding of what I've been going through. To my gorgeous nanna, Barbara. Thank you for being my best friend; thank you for being by my side through my entire life. I love you like you wouldn't believe. You mean so much to me. Thank you to my father, Reece, for supporting me through my life. Thank you for being the one person I can tell anything to. I love you. Without all these people, I wouldn't be able to get through life. You all have helped me in ways you'll never understand.

Thank you isn't enough, but thank you to Dr Tom Manley for being the only surgeon to listen to me and stick by my side for the last couple of years. Your patience with me is next level, thank you for looking after me, and going above and beyond with each surgery. Thank you for taking the time to contribute to this book and for lending us your medical brain to check we got the details right.

Thank you x 1000 to Katie Bosher, my amazing writer! Without you this book would never have come alive. You were extremely easy to work with, so easy to get along with and I absolutely loved working with you. You are an incredible person.

Thank you to the whole team at Murdoch Books for believing in my book and making my dreams come true: publishers Kelly Doust and Lou Johnson for bringing me in and getting the creative ball rolling, and Corinne Roberts for taking it to the finish line. Huge thanks to editorial manager, Justin Wolfers and editor, Alice Grundy, and to the design team: Vivien Valk, Alissa Dinallo, Susanne Geppert and Sarah McCoy. You brought everything together so beautifully.

Thank you to my agent, Ben Grand, who helped me along the way. Without your encouragement and support I would never have done this.

And finally, thank you to all my followers and community for the love and support, I love every single one of you. To every single person who picks up this book: thank you for showing your support. I really hope this book is everything you thought it would be and helps with your own journey. I'm truly so appreciative.

BONUS!!
You are not alone

Just a handful of the tons of lovely notes from my community,
that show how important it is to spread the word about endo

I started following you because of LI, but I got an endometriosis diagnosis last year and your story has helped me so much getting through it! I've had so much emotion with my bloating and always feeling horrible... I've learned a lot just from following you about different symptoms. I am sorry for what you're going through, but thank you for sharing for those of us going through similar 💕 keep spreading awareness queen!

hey erin, i just wanted to thank you for teaching me more about endo. my aunt has it and she doesn't really tell me much about it. a couple weeks ago we had to rush her to the hospital because she had another cyst. she ended up getting her fallopian tubes removed or ovaries i can't remember. but i wanted to thank you for raising awareness and you are such a strong beautiful woman and i love what you stand for. i wish you all the best and i hope all goes well for you xo

i'm so blessed to have you teach me more about endo since i had only heard of it through my aunt but i love how you spread awareness and taught me more about it. you are so strong and thankyou for everything you have done xx

If it wasn't for you sharing so much about endometriosis I would never have been diagnosed properly so thank you heaps

xxx

I just wanted to say how awesome your podcast was with Zoe Marshall. It's insane how I could relate to so many parts of your story - though I've only had four surgeries, 16 that's horrendous!!
It's such a f#cker of disease you so get used to all the crazy shit that we have to deal with and get over trying to explain it to others too. I've just started Zoladex for IVF, what a bitch that is!
It was so awesome listening to you. You've had such an incredibly rough ride with your diagnosis and surgeries yet you have a great sense of humour. You're gorgeous honest, genuine and deserve the best. X

Hey, I just want to say congratulations and how proud of you I am on sharing your journey. I often think about sharing my journey to help other people suffering with endometriosis and create even more awareness here in NZ and to share everything that comes along with it but it's scary putting yourself out to the world and it's held me back from doing so. So to write a book with such personal details is so inspiring ✨ one day I hope to be as brave as you are 💪

This is amazing Erin!! Congratulations and well done, I can't wait to read it 👏. I didn't know what endo was until I followed you and thank goodness I did as I got my diagnosis soon after. Keep spreading awareness, you're doing a great job 🖤

209

Handy resources

endometriosisaustralia.org (Australia)
endoactive.org.au (Australia)
nzendo.org.nz (New Zealand)
endometriosis-uk.org (UK)
endofound.org (USA)
verity-pcos.org.uk (UK)
pcosaa.org (UK and USA)

Help with chronic pain
The Pelvic Pain Foundation of Australia – **pelvicpain.org.au**
Pelvic Pain Support Network (UK) – **pelvicpain.org.uk**
International Pelvic Pain Society – **pelvicpain.org**
Australian Pain Management Association –
painmanagment.org.au
Pain Link Helpline (Australia) – **1300 340 357** (leave a message
with your number, and a trained advisor will call you back
for free)

Accessing your health information
In Australia you can request any health information held about you under the Freedom of Information Act. This page has all the info you need about getting this information.
oaic.gov.au/privacy/health-information/
access-your-health-information

Three Facebook support groups I love*
Endometriosis Support: a group by Endometriosis Awareness. Created January 31, 2017
facebook.com/groups/4EndoSupport/?ref=share

Endometriosis Support Group: group created July 26, 2018
facebook.com/groups/258991488034471/?ref=share

ENDometriosis: group created January 16, 2009
facebook.com/groups/21070399191/?ref=share

*Remember, there are SO many support groups online. If these ones aren't for you, keep searching until you find one that is.

References

Chapter 1: Meet endometriosis and PCOS

2. Deborah Bush, *Endo Information*, Endometriosis New Zealand, 2021, nzendo.org.nz/endo-information

3. Carlo Bulletti et al., 'Endometriosis and infertility', *Journal of Assisted Reproduction and Genetics*, 25 June 2010, vol. 27 no. 8, pp. 441–7, ncbi.nlm. nih.gov/pmc/articles/PMC2941592

4. *Treating endometriosis*, The Women's, 2021, thewomens.org.au/health-information/periods/endometriosis/treating-endometriosis

5. Australian Institute of Health and Welfare, *Endometriosis in Australia: prevalence and hospitalisations*, Australian Government, 29 August 2019, aihw.gov.au/reports/chronic-disease/endometriosis-prevalence-and-hospitalisations/summary

6. Deborah Bush, *Endo Information*, Endometriosis New Zealand, 2021, nzendo.org.nz/endo-information

7. Lucia Osborne-Crowley, A common treatment for endometriosis could actually be making things worse, The Guardian, 2 July 2021, theguardian. com/australia-news/2021/jul/02/a-common-treatment-for-endometriosis-couldactually-be-making-things-worse

8. *Ten Endometriosis Facts*, Endometriosis Australia, 2021, endometriosisaustralia.org/endometriosis-facts

9. *Woolies makes major change to grocery shopping aisle*, 7News, 25 February 2021, 7news.com.au/lifestyle/woolworths/woollies-makes-major-change-to-grocery-shopping-aisle-c-2238639

10. Endometriosis Australia, 2021, endometriosisaustralia.org

11. Funmilola M. OlaOlorun and Wen Shen, 'Menopause', *Oxford Research Encyclopedia of Global Public Health*, 19 November 2020, pp. 1–31, oxfordre.com/publichealth/view/10.1093/acrefore/9780190632366.001.0001/acrefore-9780190632366-e-176

    &

    Menopause, The Royal Australian and New Zealand College of Obstetricians and Gynaecologists, 2021, ranzcog.edu.au/womens-health/patient-information-resources/menopause

12. Jean Hailes, *PCOS – fact sheet*, 2021, jeanhailes.org.au/resources/pcos-fact-sheet

13. Ibid.

14. Jacqueline Boyle and Helena J. Teede, 'Polycystic ovary syndrome', *Australian Family Physician*, October 2012, vol. 41 no. 10, www.racgp.org.au/afp/2012/october/polycystic-ovary-syndrome

15. Ibid.

Chapter 3: Make friends with pain (not really)

17. Laura Kiesel, *Women and pain: Disparities in experience and treatment*, Harvard Health Publishing, 9 October 2017, health.harvard.edu/blog/women-and-pain-disparities-in-experience-and-treatment-2017100912562

18. Mike Armour et al., 'The cost of illness and economic burden of endometriosis and chronic pelvic pain in Australia: A national online survey', *PLOS ONE* (Public Library of Science), 10 October 2019, vol. 14 no. 10, journals.plos.org/plosone/article?id=10.1371/journal.pone.0223316

19. Ibid.

20. *Endometriosis – is it a disability?*, Endometriosis UK, 17 July 2017, endometriosis-uk.org/news/endometriosis-it-disability-37511

21. Molly Clarke, *Endometriosis & Social Security*, Centre for Endometriosis Care, October 2021, centerforendo.com/endometriosis-social-security-by-molly-clarke

22. Alli Hartley-Kong, *How has working from home affected endometriosis patients?*, 18 February 2021, Endometriosis Foundation of America, endofound.org/how-has-working-from-home-affected-endometriosis-patients

Chapter 4: Step up to the surgery buffet

24. *3.1 Tonsillectomy hospitalisations, 17 years and under*, Australian Commission on Safety and Quality in Health Care, 2021, safetyandquality.gov.au/our-work/healthcare-variation/fourth-atlas-2021/ear-nose-and-throat-surgery-children-and-young-people/31-tonsillectomy-hospitalisations-17-years-and-under

25. Dana Šumilo et al., 'Incidence of indications for tonsillectomy and frequency of evidence-based surgery: a 12-year retrospective cohort study of primary care electronic records', *British Journal of General Practice*, January 2019, vol. 69 no. 678, pp. 33–41, bjgp.org/content/early/2018/11/05/bjgp18X699833

26. Chih-Hsuan Sao, 'Pain after laparoscopic surgery: Focus on shoulder-tip pain after gynecological laparoscopic surgery', *Journal of the Chinese Medical Association*, November 2019, vol. 82 no. 11, pp. 819–26, journals.lww.com/jcma/fulltext/2019/11000/pain_after_laparoscopic_surgery__focus_on.7.aspx

27. Lucia Osborne-Crowley.

Chapter 5: My surgery survival guide

28. Department of Health, *Freedom of information (FOI)*, Australian Government, 6 September 2021, health.gov.au/about-us/corporate-reporting/freedom-of-information-foi
&
Office of the Australian Information Commissioner (OAIC), *Access your health information*, Australian Government, 2021, oaic.gov.au/privacy/health-information/access-your-health-information

Chapter 7: Painful sex – the elephant in the bedroom

29. Carli Blau, *Endometriosis and Sexual Functioning*, Endometriosis Foundation of America, 10 March 2019, endofound.org/carli-blau-phd-candidate-endometriosis-and-sexual-functioning

Chapter 10: What now?

30. Gabrielle Jackson, *Pain and Prejudice*, Sydney: Allen & Unwin, 2020, p. 272.

31. Nicola Slawson, *'Women have been woefully neglected': does medical science have a gender problem?*, The Guardian, 18 December 2019, theguardian.com/education/2019/dec/18/women-have-been-woefully-neglected-does-medical-science-have-a-gender-problem

32. Ibid.

33. Greg Hunt and Department of Health, *Funding boost for endometriosis research* (media release), Australian Government, 28 May 2020, health.gov.au/ministers/the-hon-greg-hunt-mp/media/funding-boost-for-endometriosis-research

x x x

About the author

The world best knows Erin Barnett as the hot-headed blonde who burst onto television screens during 7's *Beauty and the Geek*, before becoming runner-up on 9's *Love Island* and ultimately escaping to the South African Jungle in 10's *I'm A Celebrity . . . Get Me Out Of Here!* But behind her reality TV lifestyle lies a life full of doctor's appointments, pain medications, false diagnoses, operations, and the mental, financial and social challenges which all stem from her experience with endometriosis and PCOS.

Index